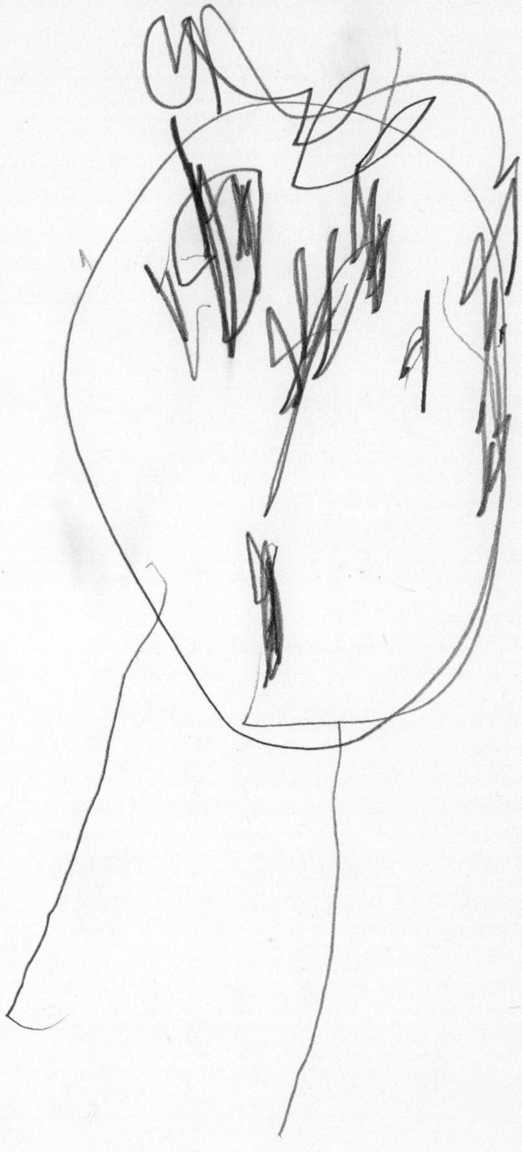

HOW TO TAKE CARE OF YOUR HORSE UNTIL THE VET COMES

A Horse Health and First Aid Guide

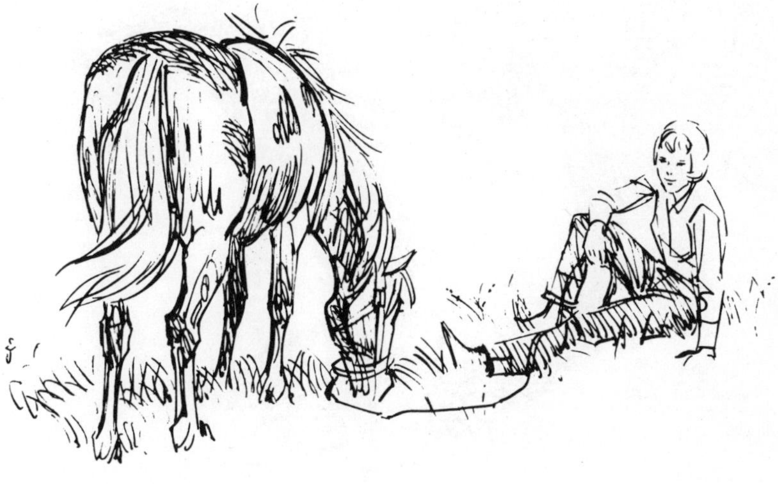

HOW TO TAKE CARE O

A Horse Health an

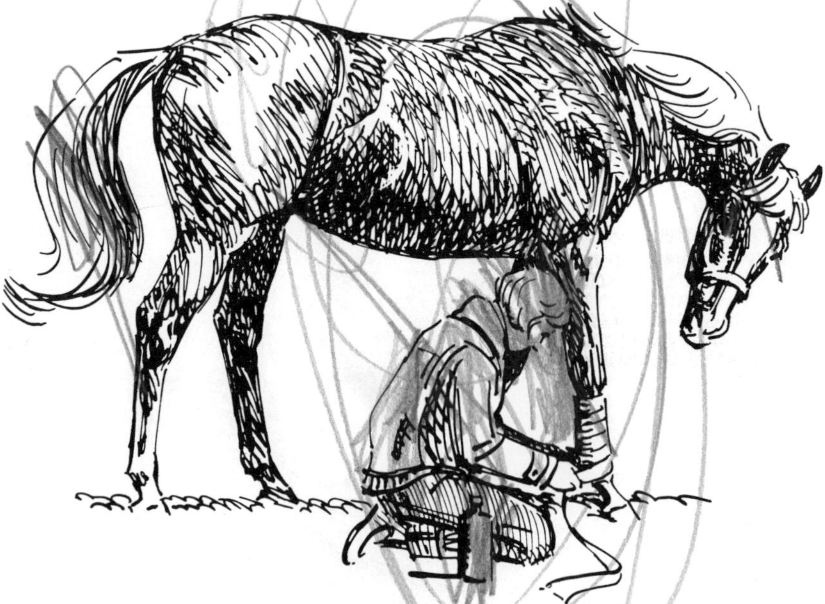

Illustrated by Sam Savitt

YOUR HORSE UNTIL THE VET COMES

First Aid Guide

HERB MARLIN and SAM SAVITT

With an Introduction by Jordan Woodcock, V.M.D.

DODD, MEAD & COMPANY NEW YORK

ACKNOWLEDGMENTS

Special appreciation must be expressed to the veterinarians who have treated our horses and graciously made themselves available to answer questions, both long before and during the preparation of this book. They include Drs. Peter Burke, Beatrice English, C. P. Gandal, Joseph A. Heissan, Joseph C. O'Dea, Ronald J. Rosen, John P. Schutz, and Jordan Woodcock.

Printed in the United States of America

2 3 4 5 6 7 8 9 10

Library of Congress Cataloging in Publication Data

Marlin, Herb.
How to take care of your horse until the vet comes.

Includes index.
SUMMARY: Includes guidelines for recognizing foot and leg ailments, internal problems, skin diseases, and injuries and gives instructions for taking temperature, reading a pulse, bandaging, and other useful procedures in both treating and preventing illness in a horse.
1. Horses–Diseases. [1. Horses–Diseases]
I. Savitt, Sam, joint author. II. Title.
SF951.M37 636.1'08'96024 75-11727
ISBN 0-396-07145-7

DEDICATED TO

the teamwork of horseowner and veterinarian in the health care of the horse

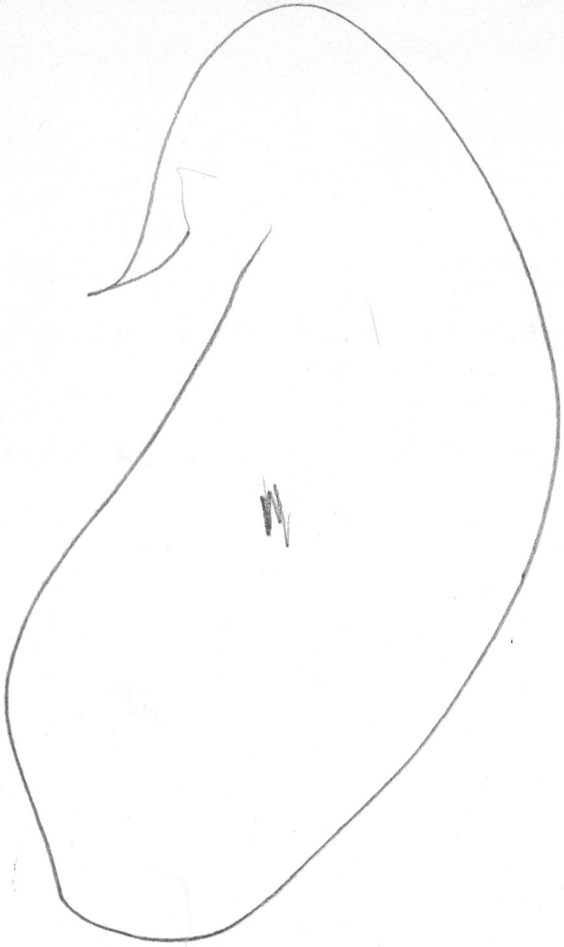

CONTENTS

INTRODUCTION

How To Take Care of Your Horse Until the Vet Comes is clear, concise, and, most important, practical. I can vouch for its practicality. It served me in a most effective manner when I used the manuscript, prior to publication, as a text for an accredited college course I was teaching. It stimulated interest in horse ailments, whetted the appetite for further investigation, and paved the way to practical teamwork between horse lover and veterinarian.

I believe my colleagues—fellow equine veterinarians—will welcome the book as an aid to their clients since it is not a "do-it-yourself veterinary book." It is unique in its call for teamwork between owner and veterinarian and its instruction on how the owner can best assist the veterinarian in the health care of the horse.

Although not pretending to be a definitive work, this book does do exactly what the title indicates—it tells and shows how to take care of your horse until the veterinarian arrives. I am happy to recommend it because your horse will benefit from it.

Jordan Woodcock, V.M.D.

Administrator of the Drug and Medication Rules of the American Horse Shows Association and a founder and former president of the American Association of Equine Practitioners

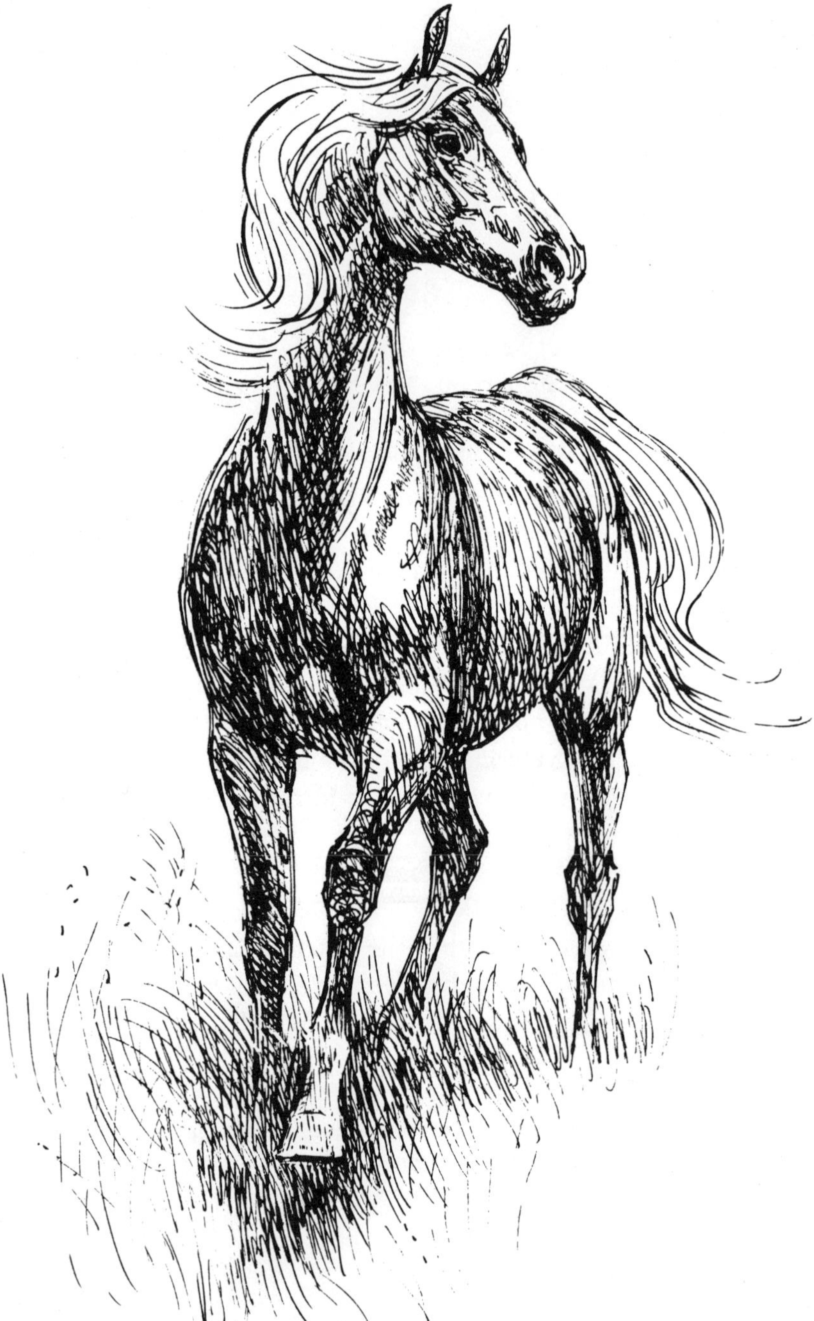

1

YOU AND THE VETERINARIAN

Be a Keen Observer — Keep a Horse Health Record — First Horse Health Goals

You and your horse's veterinarian are a team.

On the other hand, your family physician and you are not a team. If you are ill or injured, you are the patient, and your doctor has his own team of assistants.

The small animal veterinarian, with his local animal hospital to which you can bring ill or injured pets, also has a team of assistants.

Your horse's veterinarian, however, whose station wagon is his office and dispensary in the field, usually has only one assistant. That assistant is you. You can be a vital member of the medical team taking care of the health needs of your own horse. Your familiarity with your horse, your knowledge, and ability are important to the veterinarian, before he comes to treat your horse, while he is treating it, and after he leaves.

BE A KEEN OBSERVER

The best aid you can provide your horse, your vet, and yourself is to be a good observer. Know the appearance and behavior of your horse when he is in good health. It is only by knowing what is right that you can detect a condition that is wrong.

Whenever you are with your horse, ask yourself:

Is he alert and inquisitive, but not nervous?
Are his eyes bright and clear?

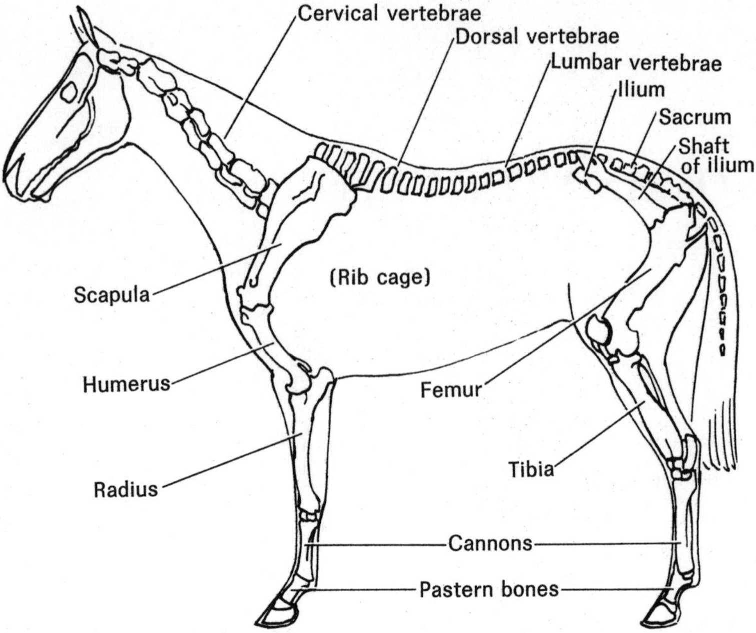

Skeleton of a horse

Is his skin glossy and pliable?
Does he move freely?
Does he stand squarely on all four feet, except when resting a hind leg?
Does he eat eagerly and finish his grain?

KEEP A HORSE HEALTH RECORD

By keeping a record of your horse's appearance and health you will be doing the veterinarian, your horse, and yourself a favor. When the vet comes and asks you questions, you will have the answers.

It is really easy. A calendar with room for brief notes makes a fine horse health record book. Note any changes in your horse's appearance or behavior. Keep track of any changes in stable management—change of feed, horse turned out, etc. If

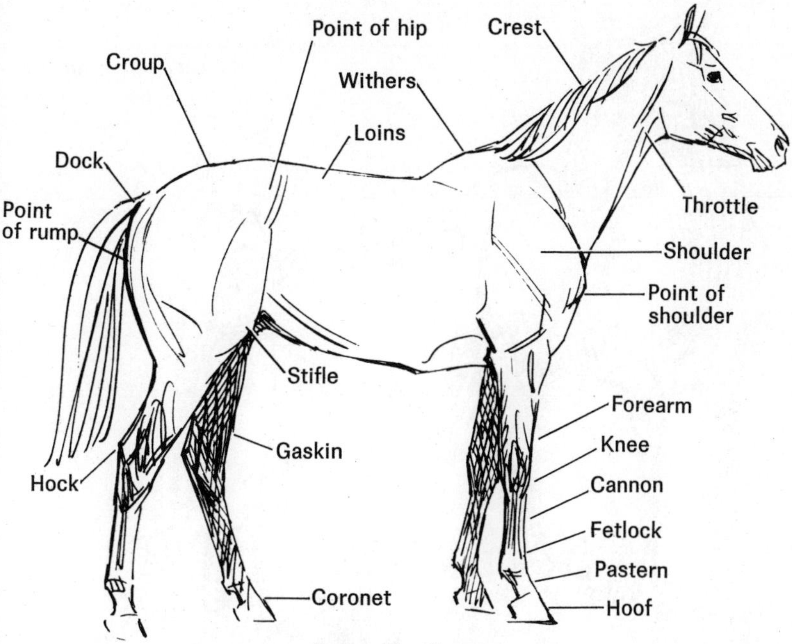

Parts of a horse

first aid is called for, note what you have done. If the veterinarian treats your horse, record what he does. Keep a record of the shots your horse gets, when he was wormed, when shod, and anything else you might need to know about exactly in the future.

Any changes in your horse's appearance or behavior should be noted, even if you don't intend to call the veterinarian at the time. You may want to call him in a few days, and it will be good to know when you first noticed the change.

It is also a good idea to keep a record of expenses.

FIRST HORSE HEALTH GOALS

If you can do the following, you will aid your horse and the veterinarian greatly:

Be able to detect the difference between your horse in good

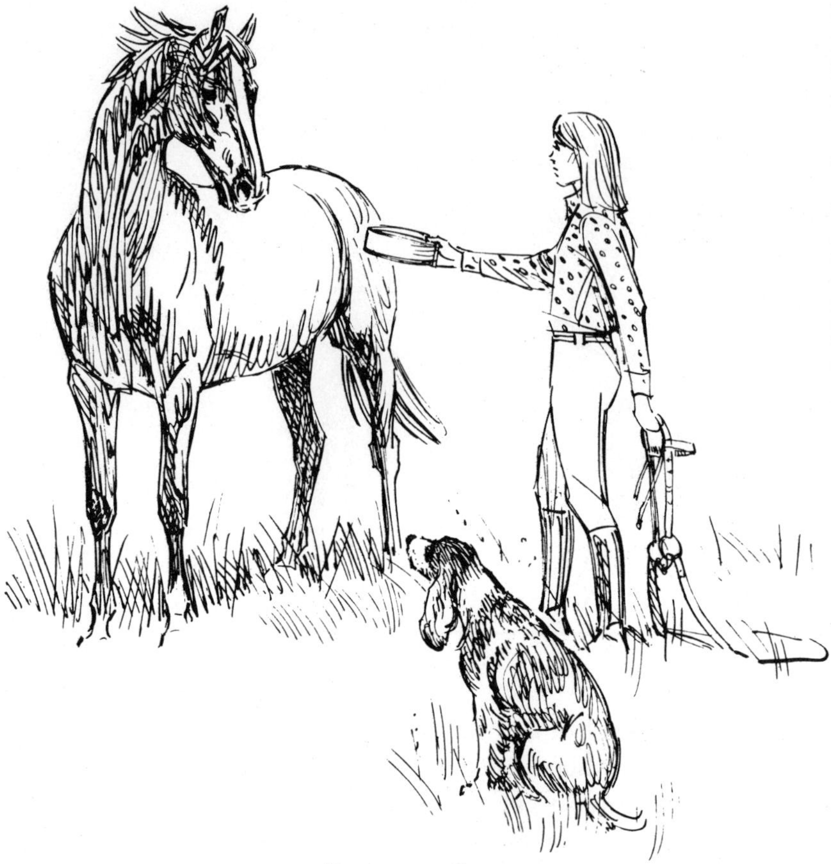

Know your horse

health and in illness.

Avoid panic when faced with injury or illness in your horse.

Keep your sick or injured horse comfortable and quiet until the vet comes.

That is a good start. But the more you know about horse health care and first aid, the more satisfying it will be to own a horse.

2

TOOLS OF FIRST AID AND HOW TO USE THEM

Taking Temperature — Reading Pulse — Checking Respiration — Removing a Shoe — Poultices — Cold Applications — Counter Irritants — Bandages — Administering Medication — Hand Rubbing and Massage — Handling the Sick Horse

TAKING TEMPERATURE

Your horse can't tell you how he feels, but his temperature can give you a good indication.

A mature horse's normal temperature is about 100° Fahrenheit. It may vary from 99° to 101°. If it goes to 102° or more, report it to your veterinarian.

When taking a horse's temperature, cross tie the animal if he stands quietly that way, or have someone hold him. An unruly horse could cause you to lose the thermometer in the horse's rectum. If that happens, don't panic. Confine the horse in its stall. The thermometer will be expelled with the horse's next bowel movement.

You will need a *rectal* thermometer. A human rectal thermometer will do, but a heavy-duty veterinary thermometer is better.

Shake the thermometer until it reads 95°F. or below. Lubricate the bulb of the thermometer with vaseline. Gently raise the horse's dock and insert the instrument in the horse's rectum. Rotate the thermometer until three-quarters of its length is

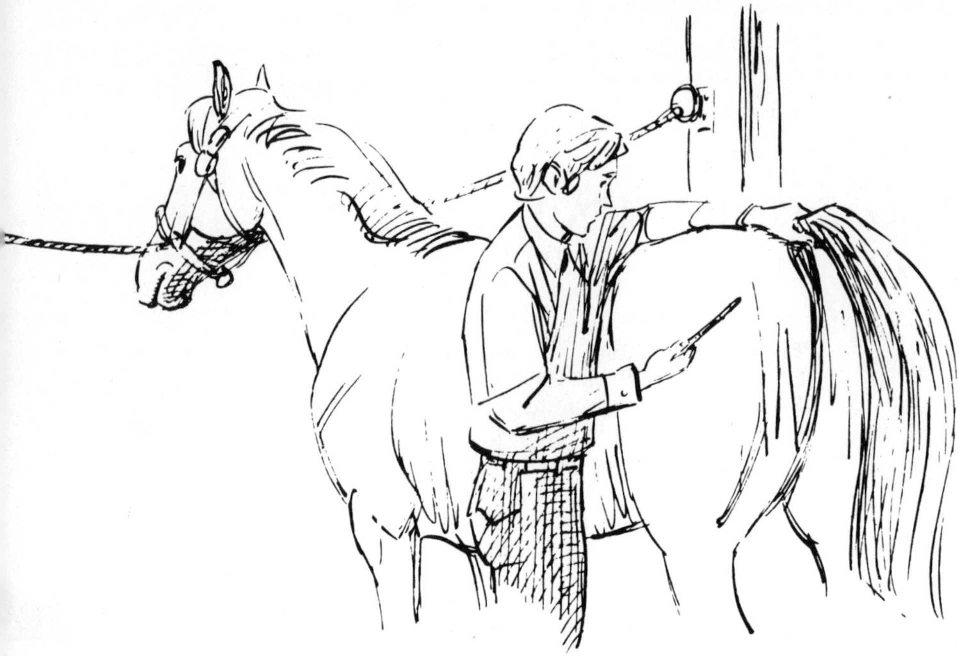

Taking your horse's temperature

within. Keep it there for three minutes, remove it gently, and you should have an accurate temperature reading.

An important suggestion: Before attempting to take a horse's temperature on your own, observe how your veterinarian does it. Ask him to check you out as you repeat the procedure. Learning from a book is good, but when using an instrument such as a thermometer on your horse, practice under competent supervision is better.

Some ABC's of Temperature and the Horse

A. If your horse is off his feed and feels quite warm to the touch, although he hasn't been exercised, take his temperature.

B. Temperature in the healthy horse varies about one degree in the course of a day. The highest point is reached in late afternoon or early evening.

C. Temperature of the horse is higher after meals and exercise.
D. Temperature in young horses is often one degree higher than in mature horses.
E. During illness, a temperature of 106° in the horse indicates great danger.

READING PULSE

Reading your horse's pulse tells you his heart rate. The normal pulse rate of a mature horse at rest averages 36 to 40 beats per minute.

The pulse may be felt underneath the lower jaw on either side. The middle finger should be applied to press the artery gently against the inner surface of the bone. You can feel the artery underneath the lower jaw, a little in front of the fleshy part of the cheek. Move your index and middle finger until you can feel the pulsations. Since the horse will probably not stand still for a full minute, count the pulsations for fifteen seconds and multiply by four. Take the pulse when the horse is at rest.

By reporting the horse's pulse as well as his temperature

Checking your horse's pulse

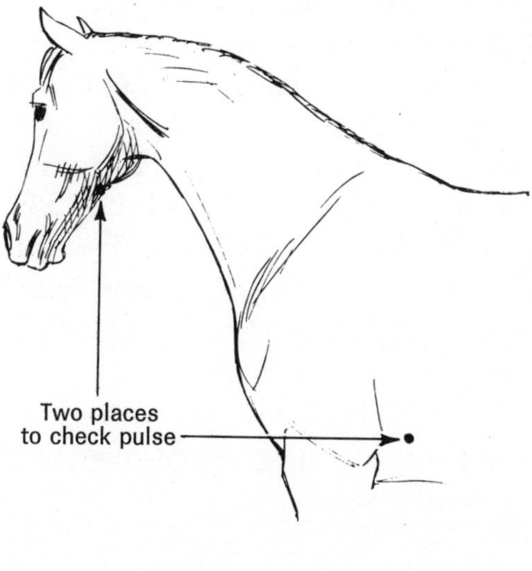

when you suspect illness, you enable the veterinarian to estimate the urgency of your call.

Some ABC's of the Horse's Pulse

A. Pulse may be taken at different locations. Underneath the jaw seems easiest for most owners. Another easy way is to place your ear against the left side of the horse's chest, just behind the elbow, and count the heart beats.
B. In reading the horse's pulse, determine if the pulse is strong or feeble, as well as its rate. This is well worth reporting to your veterinarian.
C. The pulse or heart rate is faster in young horses than in mature ones, and faster in small horses than in large ones.
D. Foals up to two weeks may have a pulse of 100; at four weeks, 70; yearlings, 45 to 60; two year olds, 40 to 50. Stallions vary between 28 and 36.
E. Excited horses show a higher rate than those at rest.

CHECKING RESPIRATION

To check your horse's breathing, watch the flank and rib cage. Each rise and fall indicates one breath. This is most noticeable in the flank just behind the rib cage. The flank and rib cage swell out when air is inhaled and fall back when the air is exhaled.

Normally, in a mature horse at rest, the number of breaths range from 8 to 16 per minute. Observing the flank and rib cage, count the number of breaths taken by the horse for 30 seconds. Double that number and you have your reading for one minute. Check your horse's respiration when he is at rest.

If your horse is not feeling well, he will be breathing much faster than normally. His respiration rate may jump to 30 breaths per minute, or even a great deal more. If that happens, report it to your veterinarian.

Some ABC's of Respiration in the Horse

A. Normally, the horse's breathing is even and regular. The nostrils move only slightly. Raising of the ribs is hardly noticeable.
B. Respiration rate is faster in young horses than in older ones.
C. Rate of respiration may be increased by activity, hot weather, overeating, lying down, or pregnancy.
D. If respiration continues at a high rate, even though the horse has rested, check pulse. If the horse's pulse is normal, don't worry. If the pulse is high, inform the veterinarian.

REMOVING A SHOE

Removal of a shoe is not for novices. Unless you have the proper tools and training, don't try it. That's what farriers are for. However, removal of a shoe can sometimes be helpful first aid.

The instructions for shoe removal and the illustrations presented here are for reference. Before you attempt to remove a shoe on your own, watch how your blacksmith does the job. Tell him you would like to know how as a first aid measure, and ask him to let you remove a shoe under his supervision and instruction.

1. When removing a shoe, remember that the last thing the blacksmith does in putting on that shoe is to turn down the nail points that penetrate the wall of the hoof. He then taps down these nail points so that the horseshoe nail becomes clinched to the wall of the hoof. The first thing then that you should do is cut the clinched nail ends on the hoof wall with a *clinch cutter*, or file them off with a *farrier's rasp.*
2. Now you are ready to use the farrier's *pulling pincers.* Hold the hoof between your knees, the bottom of the foot facing slightly upward and away from you. Grip one end of the

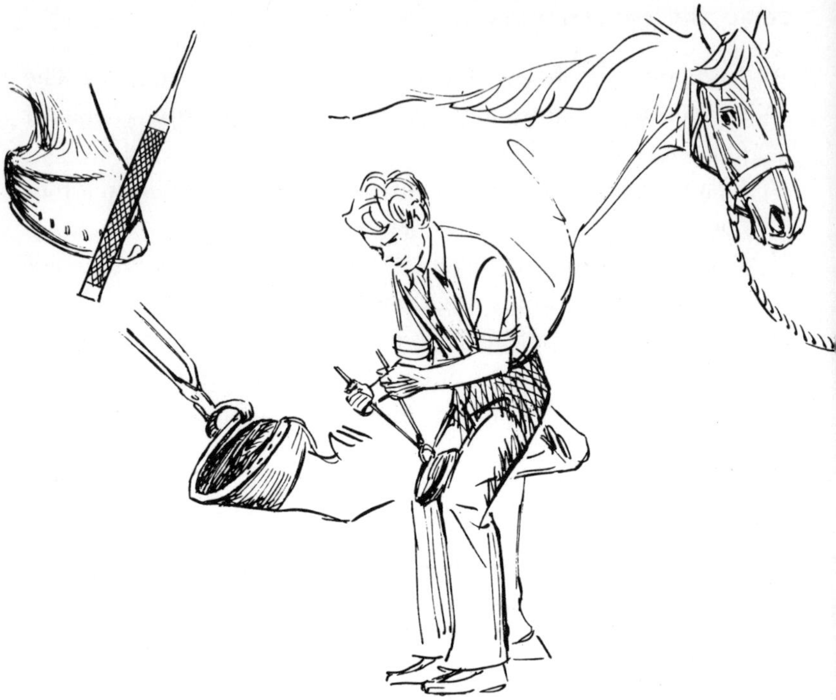

Removing a shoe

heel of the shoe with the pincers. Pry firmly but gently, loosening that part of the shoe. Keep the foot well braced and don't twist the pincers.

3. After one heel of the shoe is loosened, do the same to the opposite side. Continue gently loosening the shoe down both sides until it is free of the foot. Now check the foot to make sure all the nails have been withdrawn.

When removing a shoe, be sure to keep the foot braced, be gentle, and never twist the pincers. And never attempt to pull a shoe without the proper tools.

Save the shoe after it has been removed. When your horse's problem has been corrected, your blacksmith may be able to reset the same shoe.

POULTICES

Poultices are an important first aid tool, particularly for foot ailments. Their use makes possible prolonged application of heat and moisture to an affected part. The effect is soothing and relaxing to the tissues. The action of a poultice applied to a foot injury tends to relieve inflammation and congestion. Poultices also hasten suppuration; that is, they bring an abcess to a head so that it will burst and drain away infectious material.

The word poultice comes from the Latin *puls*, meaning porridge. Poultices are a porridge. They can be made from a variety of materials and can be bought prepared or made yourself.

Preparing and Applying a Poultice

1. Antiphlogistine is a veterinary poultice compound available at most tack shops and drugstores. It is a good, long-lasting poultice and requires only mixing with hot water.
2. Poultices can be prepared yourself from such readily available materials as bran, bread crumbs, oatmeal, flax seed, and linseed meal. (If you use bread crumbs, you will want to make sure to get rid of the salts contained in the bread. Place the crumbs in a basin and pour boiling water over them. Cover for a few minutes and pour the water off. Add fresh boiling water. The change of water will get rid of the salts.)
3. Bran is generally on hand in most stables. It makes a useful, inexpensive poultice. To make an antiseptic bran poultice, add a teaspoon of Lysol or iodine to enough hot water to dampen half a bucket of bran, and mix. Add a tablespoon of vegetable oil. Bran tends to dry quickly and the oil helps keep it moist. Mix again.
4. A commercially made rubber poultice boot simplifies applying a poultice to the foot. However, there are other ways of

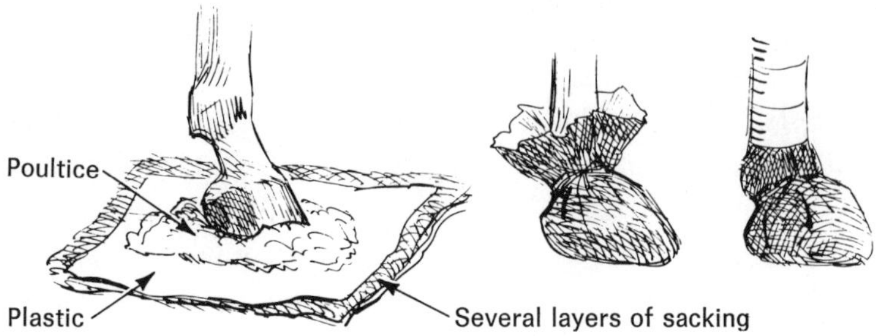

Applying a poultice

applying a poultice that will do until the vet comes. Lay several layers of sacking on the ground and a final layer of plastic material (plastic helps to retain warmth and moisture). Add the prepared poultice and get the horse to step on it. You are going to tie all this around the fetlock as you would a sack but, before you do, put a flannel bandage around the pastern so that the tying cord won't cause sore heel. It is also advisable to bandage the leg, tucking the ends of the sacking under the bandage. Foot poultices of this type slip easily. Such a poultice should be made large in order not to lose heat and efficiency quickly. Keep the poultice moist and warm, and change it daily until the vet comes.

COLD APPLICATIONS

It has been said of a well-known horse trainer that he could keep a horse racing fit with a bale of hay and a water hose. The hay was for feeding; the hose for applying cold to stressed or injured parts of the horse.

Hot or cold? Except in foot injuries, or others that may become abcessed, your first aid answer is the application of cold to injuries that do not break the skin.

The problem is to control inflammation.

Inflammation is nature's way of healing. Heat, swelling, and pain indicate that inflammation is present. This causes a larger blood flow to bring healing cells to an affected area. Too much blood, however, produces congestion. The small blood vessels rupture, and blood and fluid escape into the damaged area. This delays healing and makes complete recovery less certain.

When faced with heat, swelling, and pain, cool it until the vet comes.

Cold can be applied by a garden hose and running water, a cold stream or pool, a tub filled with ice and water, ice in cloth bags, cold compresses, commercial applications, cold water bandages, etc.

Cool it!

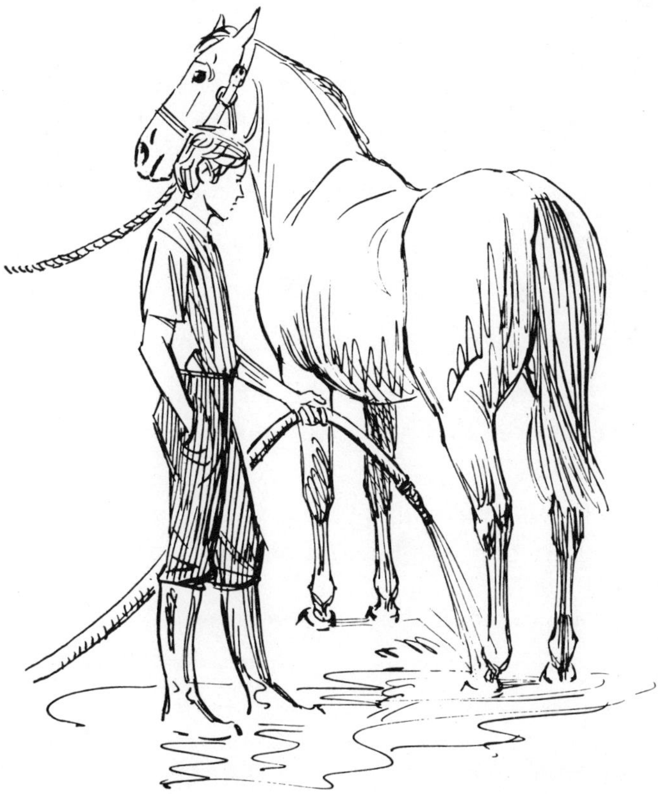

COUNTER IRRITANTS

The action of a counter irritant is the opposite of the action of a cold application. A counter irritant encourages the flow of blood to an affected area.

Counter irritants are best used after cold applications have controlled the pain, heat, and swelling of inflammation.

Liniments, various ointments, "blisters," "paints," and the firing iron all act as counter irritants.

Liniments are the mildest and safest of counter irritants. After strenuous exercise, or the stress of shipping, liniments applied with massage are good preventive medicine. They help to relieve muscle soreness in the horse as they do in the human athlete.

Ranging between the mildest and the most severe, there are many medications in both liquid and ointment form that work as counter irritants. They are available over the counter without prescription. It is wisest to use them only after an affected area has been cooled out and under the direction of a veterinarian.

BANDAGES

The main uses of bandages for the horse are:

To supply warmth to the legs and aid circulation.
To give support to joints, ligaments, and tendons while at rest or at work.
To protect legs from injury.
To retain heat or cold.
To check bleeding.
To close wounds and retain wound dressings.

Bandaging Tools

The materials needed for bandaging are available at your tack shop.

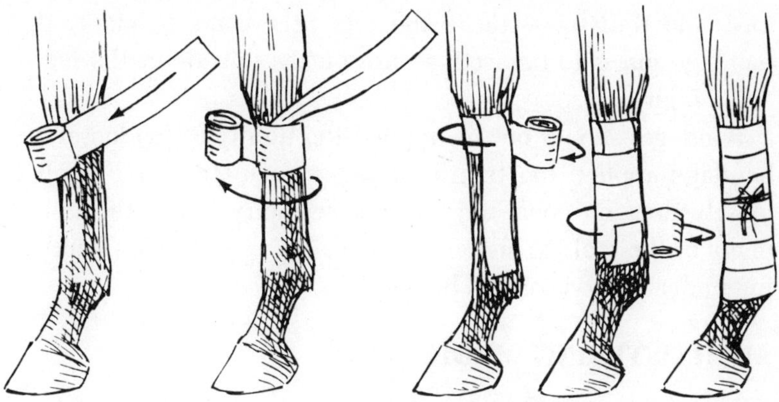

Bandaging

Leg wrappings are used under bandages. They protect the legs from air, from injurious pressure of bandages, from blows and other injuries. "Cottons" are the most frequently used leg wraps. They are made for that purpose. They are re-usable and washable, as are most bandages. There are also stitched and bound leg wraps, more expensive than sheet cottons but easier to use, particularly when medication or cold or warmth is to be applied.

Bandages have been greatly improved. Science and industry have made them more efficient and easier to apply, or "run." Although tie tapes and bandage pins are still used to secure bandages, there are some that are self-adhering or quickly secured with bandage tape. Many available bandages are elasticized, reducing the risk of interfering with circulation. There are also bandage substitutes for specific purposes, such as elasticized supportive stockings and shipping boots.

Running a Bandage

A basic standing bandage is run as follows: Over leg wraps, start the bandage rolling clockwise just below the knee or hock as illustrated. Carry the bandage down over the fetlock and pastern, and then up again to the top. Secure the bandage. If a bandage pin is to be used, secure on the outside of the leg to avoid injury.

Bandages should not be applied too tightly or too loosely. A bandage applied too tightly impedes circulation; one applied loosely does no good and may cause injury. As in the use of many of the tools of first aid for your horse, practicing bandaging under supervision can be helpful.

ADMINISTERING MEDICATION

The chief methods of administering medication available to the horseowner for purposes of first aid or nursing are internal and external.

1. Internal medication is administered through the mouth into the stomach and acts through the circulation of the blood.
2. External medication, such as liniments, ointments, lotions, etc., is applied topically or externally and acts locally.
3. Medication may also be administered by the horseowner in the form of vapor or fumes to be inhaled into the horse's lungs.

The easiest way to give medicine internally is by mixing it with the feed, either the regular grain feed or a bran mash.

The sick horse, however, may have no appetite, or the animal may refuse to eat because of the odor and taste of the medicine.

There are a few ways to trick a horse into eating feed that has been medicated. Mixing dry Jello in the feed several times before adding the medication and more Jello may disguise the odor and taste. Smearing VapoRub on the horse's nose may make it difficult for the horse to detect the medication in the feed.

The safest and best way to give liquid medicines is with a small rubber syringe. You can buy one in any drugstore. Open the horse's mouth and empty the syringe far back toward the throat without too much force.

Liquid medication may also be given as a drench. Care must be taken as drenching can be dangerous.

The bottle used for drenching should be strong, smooth about the neck, and without shoulders. A pint or quart Coke bottle will do.

Confine the animal to his stall. Back him into a corner. Have an assistant lift his head until it is horizontal as illustrated.

Introduce the bottle into the back of the mouth, in front of the molar teeth in the space called the bar where the bit lies. Elevate the bottle and pour a small amount of the liquid on the tongue as far back as possible. Remove the bottle, keep the horse's head in the same position, and encourage him to swallow by stroking under the throat latch and neck. Repeat until the prescribed amount of medicine has been given.

Care must be taken so that none of the liquid enters the lungs. If coughing occurs, lower the head immediately.

Drenching

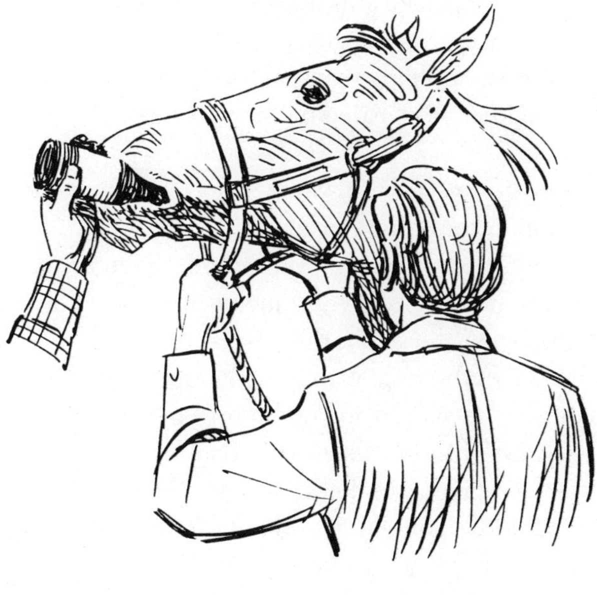

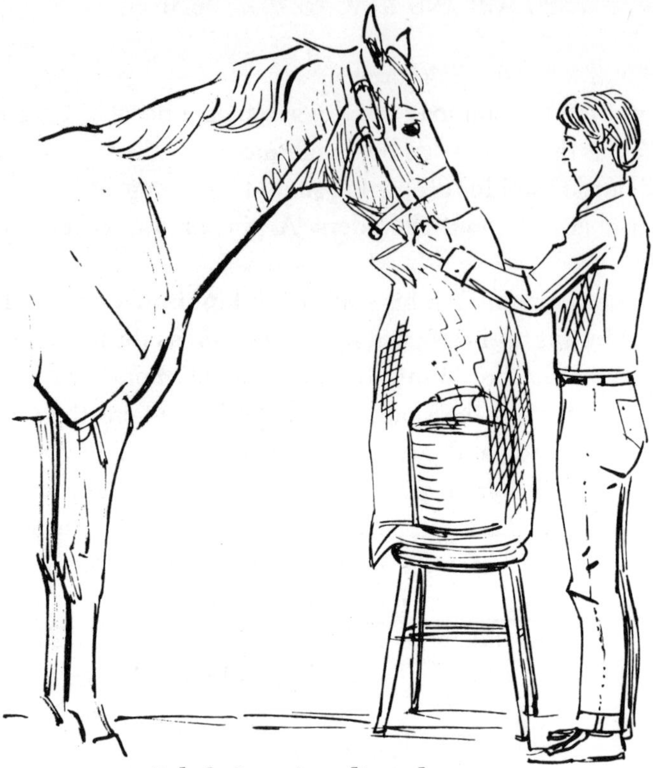

Inhalation of medicated steam

Instruction for applying external medication varies with type of medication and is indicated on the package.

Inhalation of steam with various prescribed medications is often of value in respiratory diseases.

Fill a bucket three-quarters full of boiling water, pour in the prescribed medicine, cover with hay or bran, and stir. Hold the animal's head over the steam that arises.

The bucket of boiling water, with medication and hay or bran, may also be placed in the bottom of a grain bag. Insert the horse's nose into the top of the bag so that he will inhale the medicated steam. Make sure that the steam is not hot enough to scald the animal, and do not let his head be covered.

There are curative agents used in other ways as well. These include boluses, large pills which, although taken internally, require a special instrument, a balling gun, for their administration; and injections into the muscle, into the vein, or underneath the skin. However, these are best left to the professional skill and training of the veterinarian.

HAND RUBBING AND MASSAGE

Chief aims of massage, or hand rubbing, are:

To improve circulation and aid in the removal of waste and inflammatory products.

To restore the normal functioning of an injured area by preventing or minimizing the formation of adhesions.

Massage relieves pain, increases circulation, promotes absorption, and helps prevent stagnation in the tissues.

When massaging or hand rubbing the horse, major pressure should be exerted in the direction of the heart.

Massage

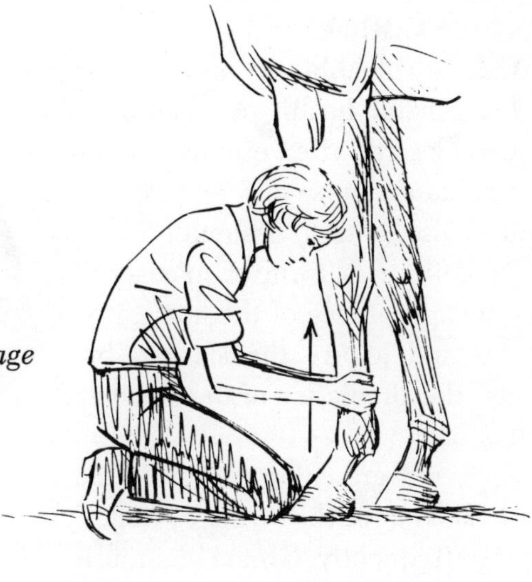

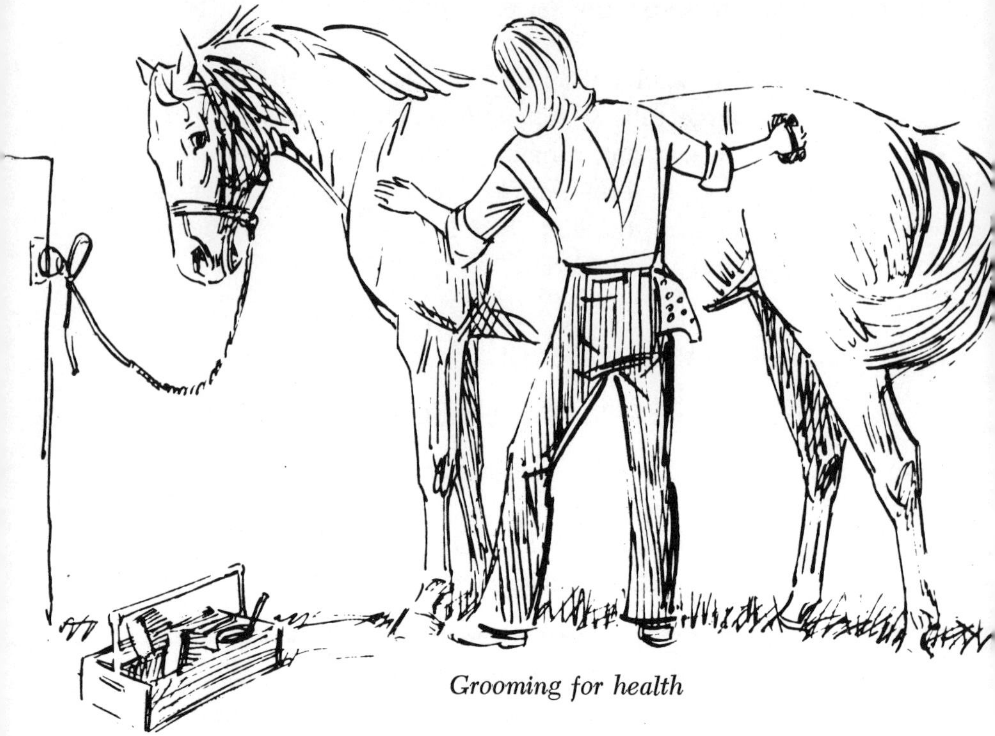

Grooming for health

In massaging the horse, start gently, and then increase firmness. To prevent irritation of the horse's skin, use a liniment or apply a little Vaseline.

Massage is valuable not only in cases of injury but also it promotes general health, as does hand rubbing. Massage is particularly useful after exercise or any other stress, such as shipping, that the horse may endure.

There is also more to grooming than meets the eye. A really good grooming is a form of massage. Grooming not only enhances the appearance of the horse, it keeps the pores in working order and allows the skin to breath. Proper grooming stimulates the circulation of the blood and promotes the healthy growth of hair.

Massage and grooming are great muscle builders, not only for the horse but for the owner as well.

Massage frequently. Groom vigorously.

HANDLING THE SICK HORSE

The first rule in handling the sick or injured horse—and all other rules stem from it—is to *keep the horse as comfortable as possible.*

1. *Stalls.* Use the roomiest stall available for the ailing horse.
2. *Bedding.* Don't stint on bedding. A good clean bed induces the horse to rest. Keep it clean and free from manure and moisture.
3. *Ventilation.* Make sure there is plenty of fresh air, but also make sure there are no drafts.
4. *Clothing.* Comfort is what you are aiming at. Use blankets according to climate. Remember that the horse can't remove his clothing when it gets too warm.
5. *Water.* Keep fresh water available at all times. The ailing horse may not drink much, but he will probably wash out his mouth from time to time, so change the water frequently.
6. *Feed.* Don't overfeed. If the horse's appetite is impaired by illness, tempt him often with small quantities of food in variety. Try a bran mash, steamed oats, chopped alfalfa, apples and carrots. If he is off his feed, the important thing is that he eat something. A little sweetened water sprinkled over the hay and grain helps. Remove anything he does not eat.
7. *Grooming.* Very ill animals should not be annoyed with unnecessary grooming. Wipe out their eyes, nostrils, and docks with a soft sponge or cloth once a day. Horses not as indisposed can be groomed normally.
8. *Exercise.* Ask the vet. The sick horse should receive as much exercise as the case permits.
9. *Avoid* noise and glaring light whatever time of day or night you visit the patient. Anything and everything that might upset the ailing horse must be shunned.

3

LAMENESS: SOME FOOT PROBLEMS AND LEG AILMENTS

ABC's of What to Look For — Corns — Bruised Sole and Frog — Quittor — Gravel — Thrush — Puncture Wounds of the Foot — Laminitis or Founder — Navicular Disease — Ring Bone — Side Bone — Osselets — Sesamoiditis — Bucked Shins — Splints — Bowed Tendon — Filled or Swollen Legs — Windgalls — Curb — Capped Hock and Capped Elbow — Thoroughpin and Bog Spavin

ABC'S OF WHAT TO LOOK FOR

A. In seeking the cause of lameness in the horse, start from the bottom—the foot—and work up to the shoulder or hip.

B. If the horse is lame in front, odds are that the cause is in the foot. If the horse is lame behind, chances are that the reason is in the hock.

C. In the stable, a horse may appear to be standing level—standing square on both forefeet—but if the pastern of one leg seems slightly more upright than the other, suspect lameness in the former.

D. If the horse points one foreleg, notice whether the heel or the toe is taking the weight of the leg. A horse generally rests the toe in laminitis or ringbone, and the heel in navicular disease.

E. In relieving an injured leg of weight, a horse uses its head position to reduce pain, raising the head as the lame foreleg comes to the ground and lowering it as the hurting hindleg comes to the ground.

F. In order to detect heat in the leg, use the back of one hand

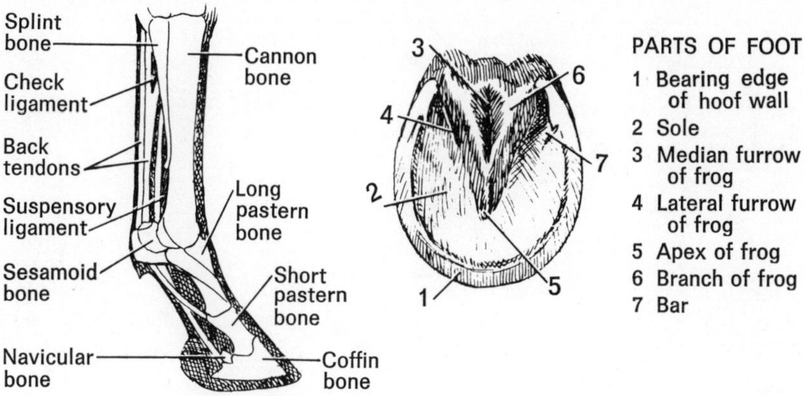

Parts of foot and foreleg

on the suspected leg and the back of the other hand on the other leg by comparison, checking every part of both legs. Any sign of heat is a danger signal.

G. Heat above the coronet, combined with pointing at rest and more marked lameness on hard ground than on soft going, indicates that the problem is in the foot.

H. In a horse that neither points nor reveals heat, and trots sound at first but then exhibits increasing lameness as work proceeds, suspect a splint.

I. If there is swelling and tenderness at the back of the leg, and lameness is more marked in soft going than on hard surfaces, sprain is very likely.

J. Sprains in the foreleg usually occur between the knee and the fetlock, and sprains in the hindleg more often will be found in the hock.

K. Elbow and shoulder lameness are frequently revealed by the horse's difficulty in bringing the leg forward in action, and also by the horse's showing pain when the limb is being carried, or the limb is off the ground. This may be due to injury, rheumatism, muscle or ligament sprains, or inflammation of the joints.

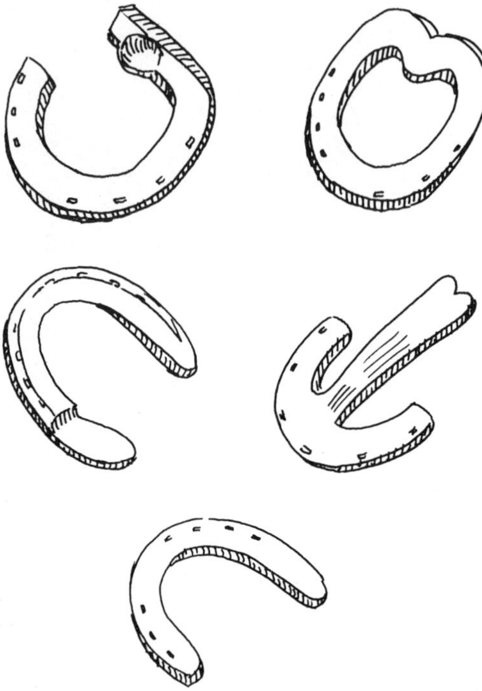

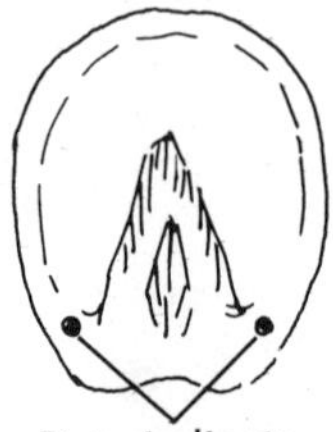

Dots indicate seat of corns

Shoes suitable for corns

CORNS

A "corn" in the horse is actually a bruise of the sensitive sole. Corns most frequently occur on the inner angle of the front feet and rarely are found in the hind feet.

Signs: Heat and pain in the foot and, frequently, extreme lameness. When the foot is raised and cleaned, you may notice a reddish discoloration at the site of the corn. If the area is tapped with a light hammer, the horse will wince noticeably.

Cause: Faulty shoeing, or a shoe that has been kept on too long. When shoes are not changed in time, the growth of the hoof carries the shoe forward. The heels of the shoe become embedded in the heels of the foot on what becomes the seat of the corn. This pressure bruising the sole causes corns.

Until the Vet Comes: Remove the shoe only if you have the proper tools and the training, and apply a hot antiseptic poultice to the foot. If you are not in a position to remove the shoe, apply the poultice to the foot with the shoe still on. The purpose of the poultice is to soften the hoof, overcome inflammation, and take out soreness.

Questions and Answers

Q. Is corn in the horse like corn in humans?

A. No. The only similarity is that both are caused by faulty shoeing. Corn in the human is an excessive growth of tissue caused by friction or pressure. Corn in the horse is a bruise or contusion—a surface injury that doesn't break the skin. The bruise causes rupturing of blood vessels, or hemorrhage.

Q. Why do corns in the horse occur more frequently in the front feet?

A. Because the front feet bear more weight.

Q. Since corn is caused by faulty shoeing, or leaving shoes on too long, can corrective shoeing help?

A. Definitely. Your veterinarian and your farrier know this well. Certain conformations of the foot may make corns more likely. Feet that are wide and flat, with heels that are low and weak, are easily bruised. Low, weak heels cause more weight and pressure on the back of the foot, and a greater tendency to bruise. Contracted heels lead to corns because the contraction works against the elasticity of the foot and increases pressure on the sensitive structures. Feet that are brittle and dry with a thin horn create a situation for the development of corns.

Q. Can proper shoeing correct these conformation problems?
A. Yes. The bar shoe is the most suitable for corn-prone horses. It is designed so that the frog takes the pressure off the affected heels.

BRUISED SOLE AND FROG

Both the sole and frog of the foot are vulnerable to bruise damage.

Signs: Symptoms are similar to corns. Tenderness, and often extreme lameness, may be exhibited. There will be heat and pain in the foot, and tapping the area with a light hammer will cause the horse to flinch. Thorough cleaning of the foot may reveal red stains indicating the bruised area.

Cause: The horse's treading heavily on a stone, on a tree stub, or wearing a badly fitted shoe.

Until the Vet Comes: If you have the tools, and the skill and training, remove the shoe. The shoe may be the chief offender. At any rate, apply foot baths and/or poultices, as either may afford some relief. Your first aid is to relieve pain.

Questions and Answers

Q. How do you apply a "foot bath"?
A. A foot bath is simple to prepare and, with most horses, easy to apply. Take a bucket and add two cups of Epsom Salts for each gallon of warm water. Place the ailing foot in the solution for at least 15 minutes at a time. Repeat the procedure a number of times during the day. Foot baths prepared with Epsom Salts (magnesium sulphate) aid in relieving the pain of bruises and act as an anti-inflammatory agent.

Q. Do I need to call the veterinarian?

A. You should, if only to get his advice. There can be complications.

Q. What sort of complications?

A. That depends on the severity of the injury. As in so many foot injuries, an abcess may develop. It should be drained by cutting away a portion of the diseased area and exposing the sensitive laminae, the susceptible leafy-like structures under the horny wall of the foot. This is a job for the veterinarian. There is another danger, depending on the severity of the injury, and that is damage to the coffin bone. Inflammation of the coffin bone (*pedal osteitis*) may be present, requiring professional care.

Q. Is corrective shoeing of any help?

A. Yes, after the horse has recovered, ask the blacksmith to

Foot bath

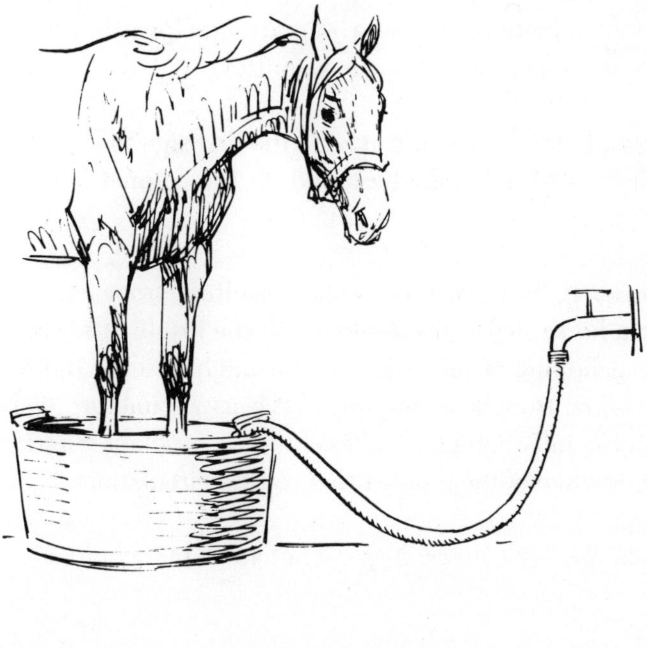

apply a wide shoe on the foot that had been injured. A wide shoe puts as little pressure on the sole as possible and will allow you to work the horse lightly. This light exercise helps bring back circulation to the bruised tissues that have become congested by the injury.

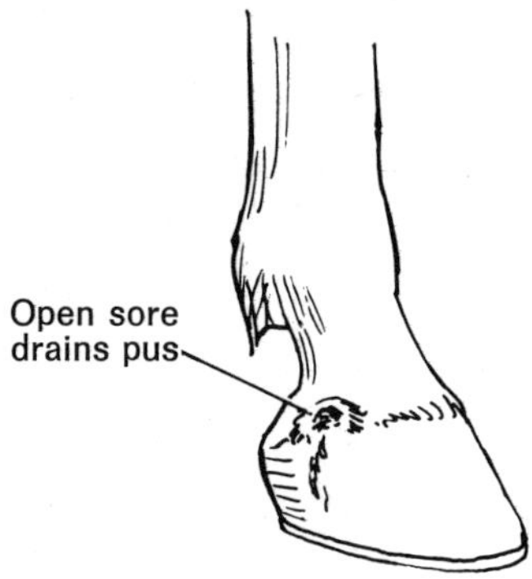

Quittor

Quittor

A foot infection causing a migration of pus that frequently shows at the coronet is known as quittor.

Signs: Painful lameness may be the first sign, but often swelling, heat, and pain may be found on the coronet before lameness.

Cause: A blow on the coronet resulting from an overreach when a horse strikes his foreleg with the inside of his hind shoe while galloping or jumping. Quittor might also be the result of some other trouble in the foot, such as a puncture wound in which the infection gains access to the coronet, or wire cuts and other damage of the coronet that reduce circulation.

Until the Vet Comes: Apply a hot antiseptic poultice.

GRAVEL

Gravel resembles quittor in that pus formation follows the line of least resistance and drainage may occur at the coronet. However, the cause is different.

Signs: Lameness usually occurs before any drainage is seen. The degree of infection and the location of the entry of infection determine the degree of lameness. Examination of the white line and sole may reveal black spots. Tapping the bottom of the foot with a light hammer can indicate the area where infection penetrated.

Cause: A crack in the white line of the foot permits infection to enter and cause inflammation of the sensitive laminae.

Until the Vet Comes: Soak the foot in an Epsom Salts bath. Again, but only if you have the proper tools and training, it would be good to remove the shoe. If it is going to be some time before the veterinarian can come, apply a hot antiseptic poultice. The sooner the veterinarian can come, the better.

Questions and Answers

Q. I always thought that the condition called gravel resulted from gravel working its way into the foot. Is that the case?

A. Old-time horsemen thought so—thus the name. But now we are reasonably sure that the cause of the infection, be it grit, gravel, or something else, finds its way into the foot because the horn is already damaged.

THRUSH

Thrush is a disease of the frog. It is found mainly in the cleft of the frog.

Signs: Most noticeable is the foul-smelling discharge that characterizes thrush. In the affected areas, black, dead tissue can be seen. Lameness may occur, but not in mild cases. This may be unfortunate, because by the time lameness does occur due to thrush, the disease already has developed to such a degree that treatment becomes difficult.

Cause: Filthy stalls, uncleaned feet, and lack of frog pressure due to poor shoeing or foot trimming all create the environment for certain micro-organisms to do the dirty work called thrush.

Until the Vet Comes: A good stiff brush and plenty of soap and water should be applied to the cleft of the frog. The stiff brush may remove loose and ragged pieces of dead frog tissue. After scrubbing the cleft of the frog, apply an antiseptic dressing. This can be one of many. Your tack shop has thrush medication on its shelves. Many race-horse trainers swear by Clorox. Lysol and other home medications have been successful. Keep the foot clean and medicated and the stall well mucked out. You may not have to call the vet. However, if signs of thrush are accompanied by lameness, do call the veterinarian.

Questions and Answers

Q. Are some horses more likely to get thrush than others?
A. Yes. Horses with high heels are especially prone to thrush.

Q. Why is that?
A. Lack of pressure on the frog, which may develop thrush even if the bedding is spotless.

Q. Why does the frog particularly require pressure?
A. Because the frog acts as a pump. It reacts to pressure like strong rubber and helps pump blood back to the heart. Not only does the pumping action aid the circulation of the

blood but it helps the glands in the cleft of the frog to be maintained in a healthy, normal state. That is why the frog requires pressure to function naturally.

PUNCTURE WOUNDS OF THE FOOT

Signs: Pain, lameness, and heat in the foot. An examination of the bottom of the foot may reveal the penetration of a foreign object or other indications that the foot has been punctured. Lameness following shoeing also points to a puncture wound.

Cause: Most puncture wounds of the foot are caused by the horse's stepping on nails, screws, or other foreign objects, or by a misdirected shoeing nail.

Until the Vet Comes: Unless such a wound gets immediate attention, symptoms multiply. Infection is carried to sensitive parts causing severe inflammatory reaction, pus forms, and pain increases. Protection against tetanus is very important in this type of wound. Get the veterinarian as soon as possible.

Do not remove the penetrating object if it is still imbedded. Let the veterinarian remove the object and treat the wound accordingly. Meanwhile, wash out the foot gently with warm water and soap and apply a hot antiseptic poultice.

LAMINITIS OR FOUNDER

Laminitis or founder is an inflammation of the sensitive structures (sensitive laminae) which lie inside the horny wall of the hoof. It is a very serious disease and acutely painful because there is no room for swelling inside the hard, unrelenting horn of the hoof.

Signs: Extreme lameness appears quickly. The feet become very hot and tender. The horse may constantly try to shift

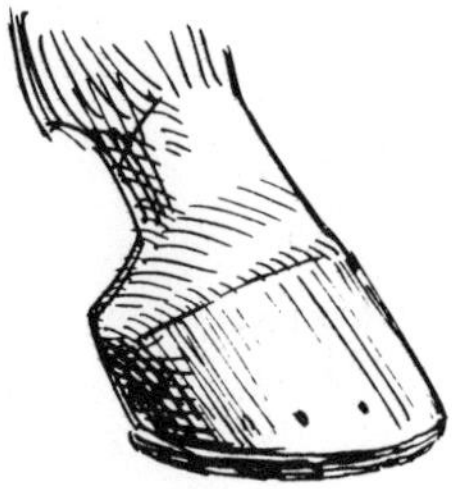

Normal foot

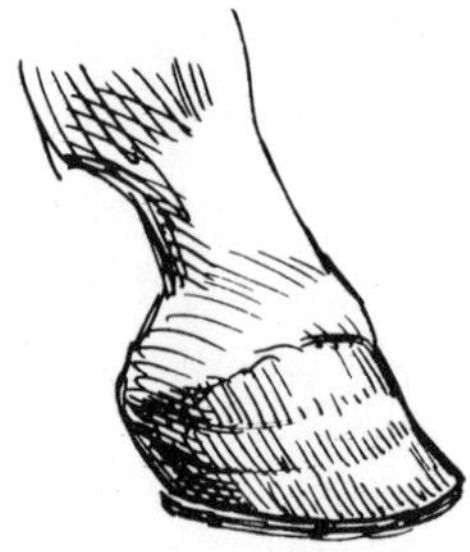

Foundered

weight in order to relieve pain, or may bunch all four feet under the body, and then stretch them out as far as possible. When walking, the horse may resemble a cat on a hot tin roof, snatching up its legs quickly to escape pain. The pulse and respiration are speeded up and temperature may reach 105° F.

Cause: There are causes, not *a* cause, and the causes at this time are not fully understood. But the following have been observed and are commonly recognized. Any of them may upset the balance of blood circulation in the feet and cause congestion, an abnormal collection of blood:

Excessive grain and lack of exercise.
Excessive work when a horse is not fit.
Excessive cold water when a horse is overheated.
Excessive lush pasture that a horse is not used to.
Excessive idleness while being fed a diet beyond maintenance requirements.

There are other suspected causes, such as hormonal influences, but those listed are the most common and agreed upon.

Until the Vet Comes: First of all, call the veterinarian the moment you suspect laminitis. Describe symptoms, pulse and temperature. Feed laxative food, bran mashes, and not too much hay. Apply cold to the affected feet.

NAVICULAR DISEASE

This is a condition of the bone of that name. Compared to its companion bones in the foot, the pedal bone and short pastern, the navicular bone is tiny. Navicular disease, however, is not tiny. Simply described, it is an ulcer eating away on the navicular bone.

Signs: When standing quietly in the stall, the horse will place one foot forward about eight or ten inches with the heel slightly raised. If both feet are affected, the horse will advance first one and then the other. When working, the horse doesn't reach out as it should and may stumble frequently. Gradually lameness develops, which may wear off with exercise or in soft going. Heat may be detected in the back of the foot. Over a period of time the foot changes shape. The heels contract and raise; the sole becomes more concave.

Cause: Anything that may tend to set up inflammation in the back of the foot may produce navicular disease. Horses that do hard and fast work are especially subject to the disease. Contracted heels and short, upright pasterns make a horse prone to navicular. Faulty shoeing, without frog pressure, can be a cause. A tendency to navicular disease may also be inherited.

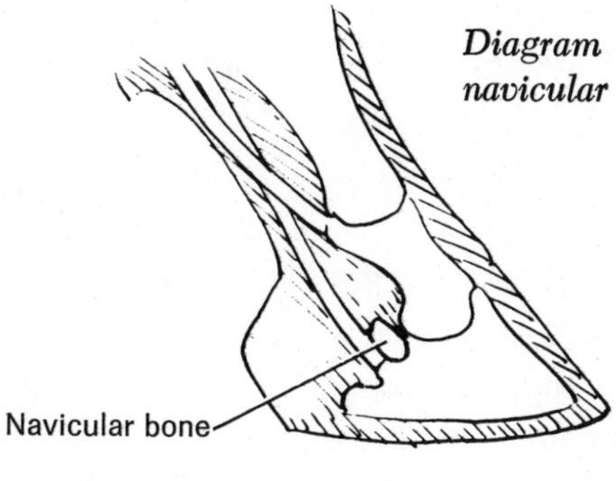

Diagram of foot, showing navicular bone

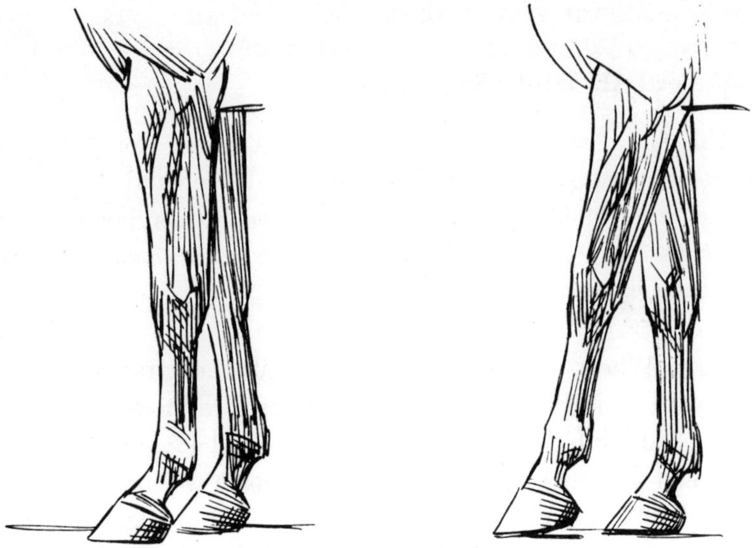

Left: *Normal stance.* Right: *Pointing may indicate navicular disease.*

Until the Vet Comes: There isn't much you can do. Cold applications to the affected area may offer some relief.

Questions and Answers

Q. What are the chances of recovery?
A. If the veterinarian's diagnosis is navicular disease, the chances of recovery are extremely poor.

RING BONE

This is the growth of new bone in a ring around the pastern. It is called low ring bone when it occurs at the top of the hoof, and high ring bone when it occurs around the pastern bones.

Signs: Lameness sometimes appears before the enlargement occurs. Since in beginning ring bone there is no heat to be felt, it is hard to trace the cause of lameness due to ring bone. In some cases an enlargement can be seen and felt before lameness occurs. After a period of a week or more, heat can be felt, and the horse evidences signs of pain.

Cause: This bony enlargement, like others, results from inflammation of the enveloping membrane of the bone due to:

Concussion, particularly when too straight pasterns cause excessive jarring.
Injury and infection, especially wire cut wounds.
Poor shoeing, or irregular shoeing, allowing the heels to grow too long, removing frog pressure and increasing concussion on the foot.
An inherited tendency to ringbone.

Until the Vet Comes: Apply cold treatment. First aid practice has shown that it is desirable to put the horse on a laxative diet. Leave the rest to the veterinarian.

Questions and Answers

Q. What is the enveloping membrane of the bone?
A. It is a skinlike covering of the bone, a fine sheet of specialized tissue. The scientific term is periosteum.

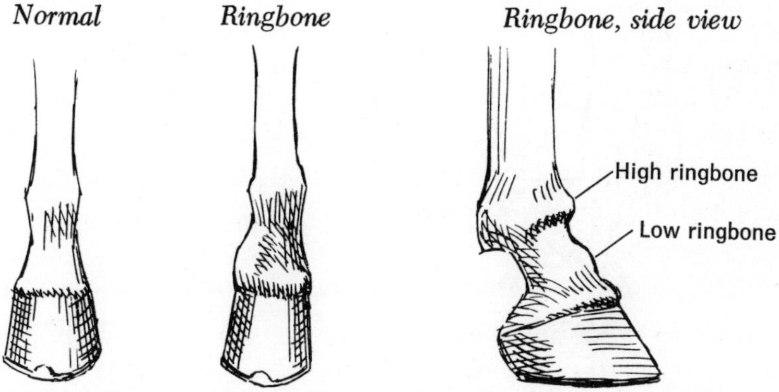

Q. What are the chances of recovery from ring bone?

A. If it is observed early, and the joint is not involved, chances of recovery are good.

SIDE BONE

Side bone is similar to ring bone. Its appearance is different in that the bony enlargements are on the sides of the foot and do not meet in front, and sometimes only one side is enlarged.

Signs: A hard lump and heat can be felt on the coronet on either side of the foot. Lameness may or may not be present. Lameness, however, is rare.

Cause: Concussion of the quarters of the foot injuring the cartilages is probably the cause in most cases. It is possibly hereditary since conformation faults such as narrow feet predispose the horse to side bone.

Until the Vet Comes: Treatment is not necessary if the horse is not lame. If the horse is lame, rest him until he can be examined and perhaps X-rayed by the veterinarian.

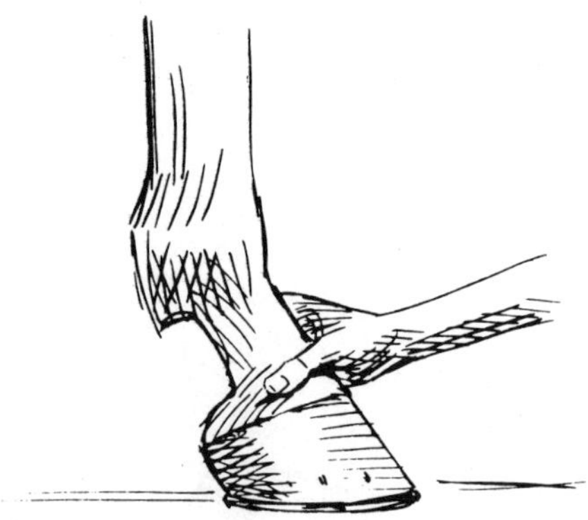

Feeling for side bones

OSSELETS

Osselets are bony growths on the fetlock or ankle joint resulting from inflammation of the enveloping membrane of the bone. They are most common in young race horses, although hunters and other horses called upon to train and compete athletically are susceptible.

Signs: The horse's gait becomes short and choppy. The horse may show signs of pain if you manipulate the fetlock joint. Examination around the fetlock joint may reveal a soft, warm, and sensitive swelling. This soft swelling of fluid and tissue can become a bony outgrowth.

Cause: Concussion and both fast and heavy work are probably the major causes. Injuries such as wounds, bruises, and strains are other causes.

Until the Vet Comes: Rest the horse. Excessive stress may have caused the problem in the first place. Apply cold treatments. If caught early (green osselets) and the veterinarian is informed, chances of recovery are quite good.

SESAMOIDITIS

This is an inflammation of the bones situated just above and below the fetlock joint, the proximal sesamoid bones.

Signs: Pain and swelling of the fetlock joint. The horse will be lame, seem to recover, and become lame again. Heat in the joint may also be on again and off again. Pressure on the joint will cause the horse to flinch. In some cases the horse will not bring the heel of the shoe to the ground.

Cause: An unusual strain in the area. Although sesamoiditis can affect any type of horse, it is most common among horse athletes, such as hunters, jumpers, and race horses. Conformation faults such as upright pasterns and turned out toes make a horse prone to the injury.

Until the Vet Comes: Rest the horse. Cold applications should be used to reduce inflammation.

Questions and Answers

Q. What are the chances of recovery in sesamoiditis?
A. In spite of a number of methods of veterinary therapy, veterinarians are not too optimistic. In other words, "The prognosis is guarded to unfavorable." Frequently, in sesamoiditis, the suspensory ligament is affected.

Q. What is the suspensory ligament?
A. Ligaments tie bones together. They consist of tough connective tissue, binding bones where they join. The suspensory ligaments referred to in sesamoiditis come down from behind the knee, then around the sesamoids, providing a supporting band to the fetlock joints. The attachments fasten to the extensor tendon in front of the limb. The sesamoid bones can be described as pulleys for the suspensory ligaments.

Q. What happens when the suspensory ligament is affected?
A. The sesamoid bones and the suspensory ligament, which function to support the fetlock under great stress, sometimes fail.

Q. Is this connected with what is called "breaking down" in a hunter or a race horse?

A. Yes. Any horse that undergoes great stress—the barrel racer, calf-roping horse, and others including the hunter, jumper, and race horse—is subject to the accident and injury commonly referred to as "breaking down." The suspensory ligament may be broken or forcibly torn (ruptured) either above or below the sesamoid bones. The result is that the fetlock and pastern joints lose their support. The accident occurs most often in a tired or unfit horse, when the muscles fail to support the ligaments.

BUCKED SHINS

Sometimes referred to as sore shins, bucked shins is another case of inflammation of the enveloping membrane of the bone —in this instance, the cannon bone.

Signs: The front of the cannon bone becomes swollen. The swelling is warm to the touch and, if pressure is applied, the animal will show signs of pain. The swelling becomes thick and looks "bucked" in front of the cannon. The horse will be lame

Normal

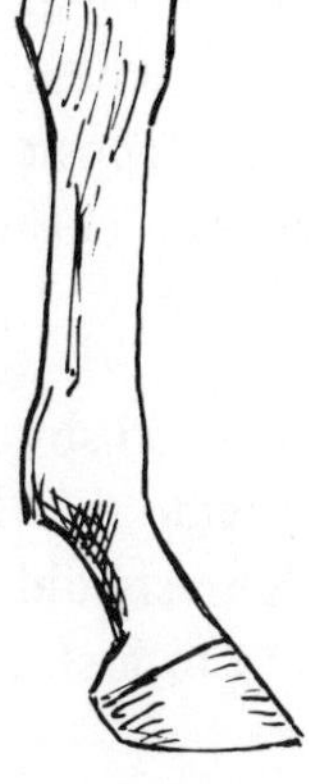

Bucked shins

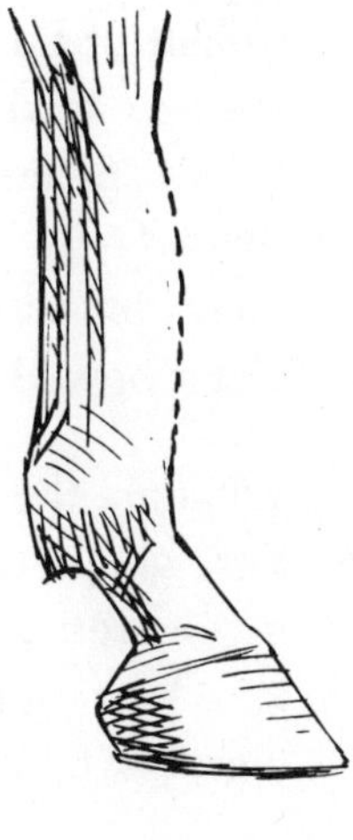

and "ouchy." If only one leg is involved, the horse will shift its weight from one leg to the other.

Cause: Hard workouts or galloping on a hard surface. It is most common in young race horses early in training.

Until the Vet Comes: The best thing you can do is rest the horse. Rest will heal most cases. Cold treatment, for the first day or two, or until the vet comes, will cool out the leg and prepare it for whatever therapy the veterinarian deems advisable.

Questions and Answers

Q. Is bucked shins an ailment that affects only young horses?
A. No, but it is primarily an affliction of young horses in hard training. The shin or cannon bone of the young horse is softer than that of a fully grown horse. It is still growing.

Q. What happens inside the leg in bucked shins?
A. The shin or cannon bone, like all other bones, has an enveloping membrane or sheath. Two tendons bear against this membrane; you might even say they rub against it. This is the road to severe inflammation of the membrane. The weight of horse and rider, the concussion they cause, and tendons working or rubbing against the membrane, cause severe inflammation. This creates a weakness that nature combats by throwing out a calcium deposit. Sometimes these deposits are small. Most times, the entire shin bone seems bowed forward, or "bucked."

Q. What are the chances of recovery in bucked shins?
A. Very good. Your veterinarian will provide the therapy, and if you are careful to rest the horse, there should be no problem. Resting the horse is the key, both to first aid and nursing after-treatment.

SPLINTS

A splint is a bony growth on the side of the splint bone that is found more often on the inside of the leg than on the outside. This is another case of calcification of the bone. Splints most often appear in young horses. The bony growth is seldom thrown out after a horse reaches full maturity.

Signs: Even if there is nothing to be felt at the time, the horse may go suddenly lame, the lameness increasing with exercise. The horse may walk sound and trot quite lame. When a splint is suspected, the best way to find it is to pick up the foot and press your fingers down the splint bone until the horse flinches. The worst position for a splint is high up and under the knee.

Cause: Severe jarring of a young horse's legs. Bad conformation of the legs and feet is conducive to splints, as is too much pressure being brought to bear on the outside of the foot by faulty shoeing.

Until the Vet Comes: Rest the horse and treat the leg with cold applications.

Questions and Answers

Q. When the splint becomes visible, what does it look like, and how big does it get?
A. It can look like, and be as big as, anything from a pea to a walnut.

Q. What are the splint bones?
A. The splint bones, placed alongside the cannon bones, are remnants from the prehistoric horse. They are reminders

that the horse once had five toes instead of the one he now stands on, tiptoed and always ready to run. These remnants of the prehistoric horse may seem useless troublemakers but they still have some anatomical purpose. They help to support the numerous bones of the knee and hock.

BOWED TENDON

A bowed tendon results from a rupture of the sheath which encloses the tendon running from knee to fetlock joint, the flexor tendon. This rupture causes excessive fluid in the tissues (edema) and internal bleeding (hemorrhage). It is a severe sprain.

Cause: Extreme exertion in the hunt field, over jumps, on the race track, or in rodeo events when a horse is tired or not sufficiently conditioned. Conformation faults such as pasterns that are too long, or crooked legs tied in below the knee (circumference of cannon just below knee noticeably smaller than rest

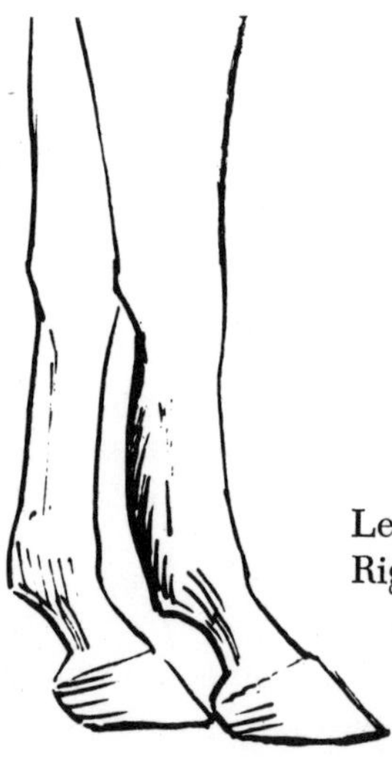

Left: *Normal*
Right: *Bowed tendon*

of cannon), may make the horse more vulnerable to bowed tendons.

Until the Vet Comes: Rest the horse and apply cold to the affected area. Until the veterinarian comes there is not much more you can or should do.

Questions and Answers

Q. What are tendons?
A. They are tough cables that connect muscle to bone and transmit the horse's power to its legs.

Q. If tendons are so tough, why do they become injured?
A. In most instances a sprained tendon is due to a rupture, a break or tear, of the ligaments that attach the tendon to muscle or bone. The tendon itself is rarely strained, sprained, or stretched. But once a tendon is stretched, it remains that way. It does not have the ability to retract, the way a rubber band or a ligament might.

Q. What are the chances of recovery from bowed tendon?
A. Not too good. A bowed horse, when he is asked for effort, may rebow.

Q. Would you say chances of recovery from bowed tendon are hopeless?
A. No. The degree of severity in tendon injuries determines the horse's chances. Flexor tendons run all the way from the top of the knee to the toe. The location of the bow determines the severity of the injury. A low bow above the fetlock offers a better chance of recovery than a high bow. When the bow is high, and involves the check ligaments at the top of the knee, chances are not good.

FILLED OR SWOLLEN LEGS

Signs: A horse's legs may become puffy and swollen if he is left standing in the stall after considerable work. This kind of swelling "fines down" if the horse is let out and exercised.

Cause: The wear of work and resulting congestion of blood in the legs.

Until the Vet Comes: Hand rub the legs, exerting pressure toward the heart. Apply pressure bandages. These should extend from below the knee to the coronet. Unless you suspect that sprain or injury is causing the swelling, the veterinarian need not be called.

Questions and Answers

Q. In hand rubbing legs, why is the pressure directed toward the heart?

A. By exerting pressure toward the heart in hand rubbing and massage, you are aiding circulation. The leg is nourished by blood brought to it by the arteries. The blood returns to the heart by way of the veins and in doing this it has to travel against the force of gravity. It does this partly through the pumping pressure of the heart and by the massaging action on the veins by the muscles and tendons when the leg is in action. By hand rubbing toward the heart, you are aiding the heart, muscles, and tendons in returning blood to the heart, and draining fluid from the limbs.

WINDGALLS

Windgalls or wind puffs are small, puffy swellings on each side of the tendons just above the fetlock.

Signs: The swellings are soft, made up of fluids, and can be pushed around. Lameness is rare.

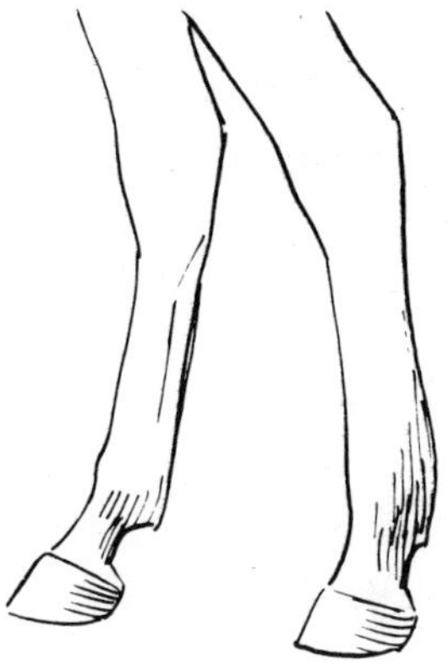

Left: *Normal*
Right: *Filled or swollen*

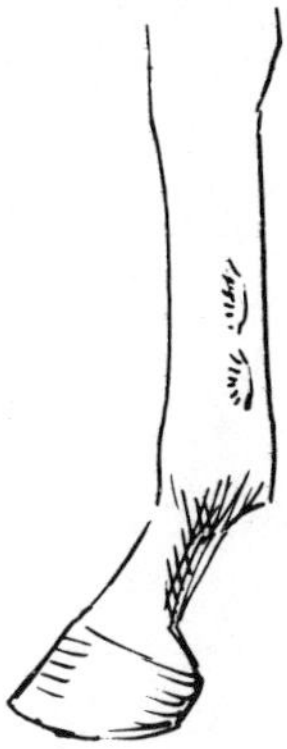

Windgall or wind puff

Cause: Young horses under heavy training will almost always develop windgalls. Race horses, rodeo horses, and show horses getting heavy work will develop them. Nutritional deficiency may make a horse particularly prone.

Until the Vet Comes: No first aid is recommended unless there is lameness, and there is no need to call the veterinarian. Decrease the work of the horse. Windgalls usually disappear. Bandaging hastens recovery. If there is lameness, call the vet.

It may be comforting that windgalls seem such a minor and harmless ailment, but remember that any abnormality, any deviation from the norm, is a warning from nature. In the case of windgalls, nature may be telling us that an adjacent structure is beginning to wear, a cartilage in the fetlock joint has been bruised, or, perhaps, a joint has been twisted. Pay attention to nature's warnings.

CURB

A curb is a sprain of the tendon or ligament at the back of the hock.

Signs: There is a noticeable swelling on the back surface of the rear cannon, about four inches below the point of the hock. Heat may be detected. If there is any lameness, the horse will go on its toe. While standing, the animal will raise the heel off the ground.

Cause: Anything that brings about overexertion of the hock. Curb may be brought on by straining in poor going, and jumping in rough country. Young jumpers are particularly prone. Curb may also result from injuries in the stall or trailer, due to kicking stall walls or trailer gates.

Until the Vet Comes: Cool out the area with cold applications. If the area feels cool to the touch before the veterinarian arrives (it will probably take three days for the area to cool out), apply a counter irritant, preferably one in ointment form.

Questions and Answers

Q. Do conformation faults in the horse contribute to curbs?
A. Yes. Horses with sickle hocks or cow hocks are particularly prone.

Q. Is corrective shoeing of any help?
A. After a horse has been rested, treated, and is ready to return to work, a high, wedge-heeled shoe can help.

Q. What are the chances of recovery in curb?
A. The chances are good if the horse has good conformation. If the horse's conformation is poor, the chances are poor because the cause is still there.

CAPPED HOCK AND CAPPED ELBOW

Capped hock is a swelling that occurs on the point of the hock. It is a bruise, and the result of injury to the hock in the hind legs, or, in the case of capped elbow, a similar injury to the elbow in the fore legs. Capped elbow is sometimes called "shoe boil" because the shoe of the affected leg may have caused the injury during motion, or while the horse was lying down.

Signs: The blemish is usually quite noticeable. It may be as large as a walnut or an orange, or may be quite small and escape notice without careful examination. Lameness is not usually present. If lameness is present, it is quite mild.

Cause: Injury resulting from poor bedding, hard and uneven floors, riding the tailgate of trailers, kicks, falls, and being rubbed by the heel of a shoe while lying down.

Until the Vet Comes: Apply cold applications immediately.

Questions and Answers

Q. Can the blemish resulting from capped hocks or elbows be removed?
A. If the cause is removed, and if the veterinarian treats the case before extensive growth of connective tissue (fibrosis) occurs, the chances are good.

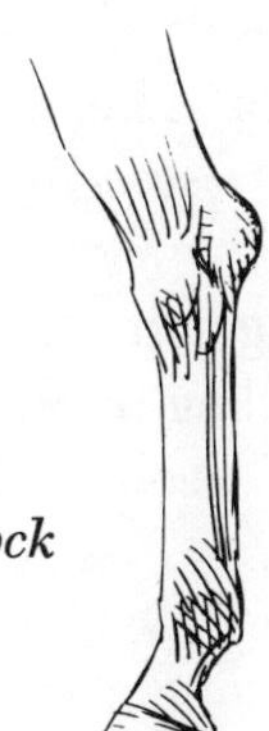

Capped hock

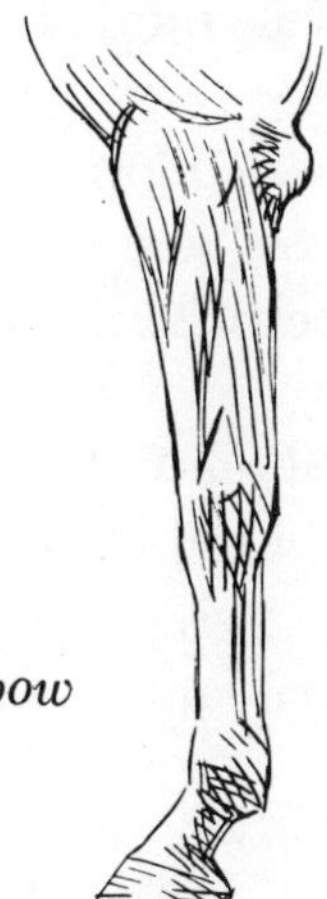

Capped elbow

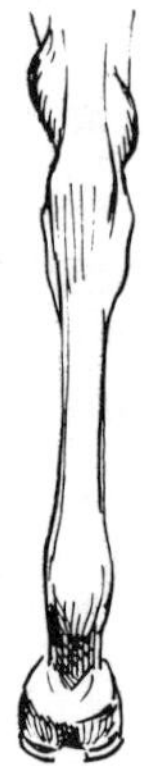

Thoroughpin

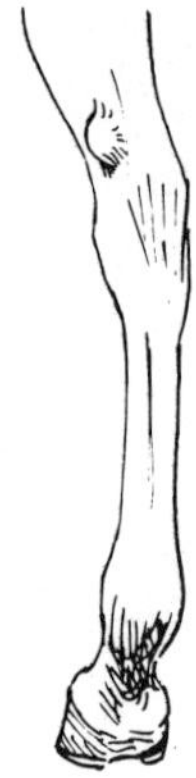

Bog spavin

THOROUGHPIN AND BOG SPAVIN

These are both found in or around the hock. Thoroughpin is the distension of the sheath of the deep flexor tendon above the point of the hock, and bog spavin is the distension of the capsule of the hock joint.

Signs: In thouroughpin there is puffiness on the upper and back part of the hock. If you press the swelling on one side of the hock, it will bulge out on the other side. Bog spavin can be seen as a swelling on the inside of the front of the hock and about one third of the way down the hock.

Cause: Injuries to the hock joint resulting from quick stops and turns, and conformation faults such as being too straight in the hocks. Nutritional deficiencies are also considered a cause.

Until the Vet Comes: If the swelling is small and there is no sign of heat, leave it alone. If the swelling is large with heat or lameness, rest the horse, apply cold treatment, and call the veterinarian.

4

SOME INTERNAL PROBLEMS

Colic — Worms — Tie-up or Azoturia — Colds — Equine Influenza or Shipping Fever — Strangles — Congestion of the Lungs — Pneumonia — Pleurisy — Congestion of the Kidneys — Staggers — Thumps

COLIC

Colic in the horse resembles a "bellyache" in humans. Because of the nature of the horse's stomach, it can be much more dangerous in equines. Colic may only be a mild intestinal discomfort, or it may come on suddenly and painfully, leading to complications that can cause death. It is more common in horses than in other animals. Most horses will suffer an attack of colic at some time or other.

Signs: The discomfort and pain that colic causes the horse to suffer are quite apparent. The horse may show any or all of the following symptoms:

Restlessness, with pawing and stamping of the feet.
Turning and looking at the flanks, the site of the pain, and kicking at the abdomen.
Lying down, rolling, and sweating profusely.

At the sign of any of these symptoms, call the veterinarian immediately.

Cause: Poor and irregular feeding and watering. However, even the best-managed stables may be faced with attacks of colic. Some horses are particularly prone to colic and have repeated attacks. "Cribbing" (chewing on wood and sucking in wind) makes a horse colic-prone and may even cause colic. The fact that horses frequently suffer from intestinal worms is another important factor leading to colic.

Until the Vet Comes: Place the horse in a roomy, well-bedded box stall. Wring hot water out of regular absorbent blankets (not horse blankets) and wrap around the belly and flanks, or roll up a hot blanket and apply it to the belly. This relieves pain and encourages the action of the bowels.

If the horse wants to lie down, let him. But if he throws himself down violently, endangering internal organs, get him up, blanket him, and walk him. Hopefully, walking him around will help to dispel gas.

Drench the animal with colic medication that your veterinarian may have prescribed earlier. If you do not have specific colic medication, make a drench with an ounce of whisky mixed with an ounce of water and administer that. Repeat in twenty minutes if the horse is still in distress. A drench consisting of two tablespoons of bicarbonate of soda mixed with two-thirds of a quart of warm water may also afford the horse some relief. Check emergency measures with your veterinarian when you call him, and carry out his instructions.

Questions and Answers

Q. Why is colic more common in horses than in other animals?

A. The frequency of colic in the horse is due mainly to the nature of the equine digestive system. The horse's digestive system is unlike that of other animals and humans. The equine stomach and its digestive surface is extremely small. The intestines, on the other hand, are extremely long, with many twists and turns and extreme differences of diameter.

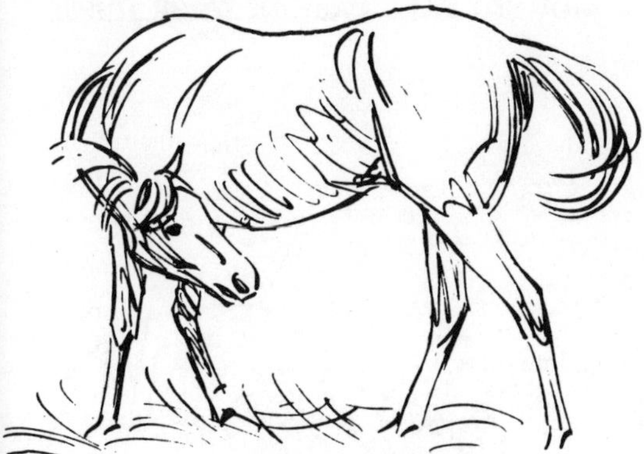

Looking at abdomen

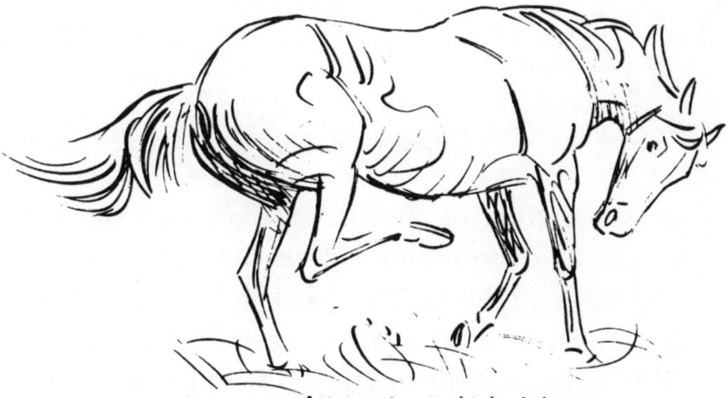

Attempting to kick abdomen

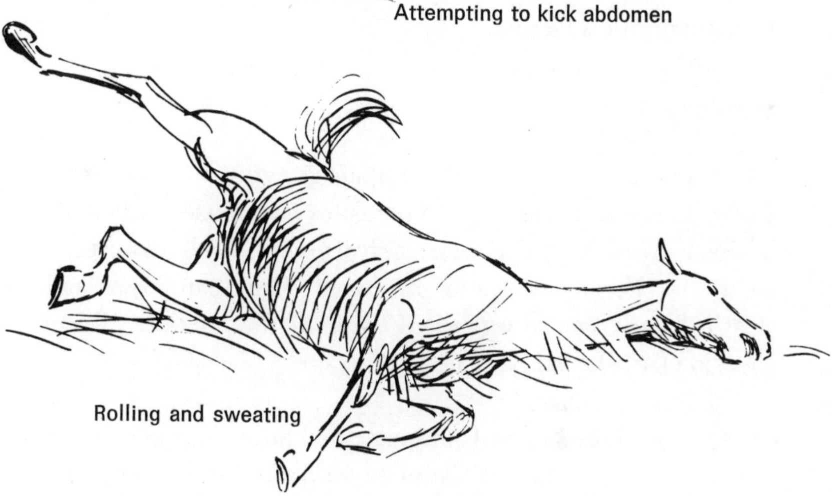

Rolling and sweating

Symptoms of colic

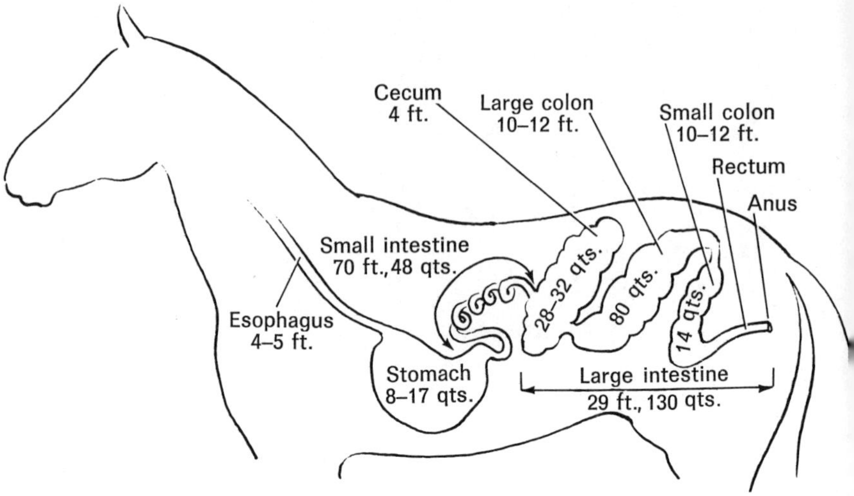

Digestive system of a horse

Any variation of the normal flow of food through these twists and turns, and sudden tight squeezes, may cause a digestive problem. The facts that the horse cannot truly vomit when something disagrees with its digestion and that it is so susceptible to internal worm damage are important contributing factors.

WORMS

Worms or internal parasites impair growth, development, and performance in horses. These parasites can cause inefficient use of feed, anemia, blood vessel obstruction, lung damage, and injury to the stomach and intestines. They can even lead to death. Nearly every organ and tissue of the horse is subject to invasion by internal parasites.

Signs: Rough coat, tail rubbing, weakness, poor performance, cough, and colic may all point to worm infestation.

However, and this is most important, a horse may be heavily parasitized and not show any external signs.

Cause: The major cause is the horse's basic susceptibility to worm infestation. Almost every horse has some worms. The problem is to keep them in check. Contributing causes are poor sanitation, manure not properly disposed of, and contaminated feed, water, and pasture.

Until the Vet Comes: Practice good stable management and sanitation before the veterinarian comes and after he goes. Protect feed and water from contamination. If possible, rotate pasture to break up worm cycles. Provide the veterinarian with several specimens of manure for microscopic examination so that the type and number of worms can be identified. In this way he can determine the proper drug or vermifuge to use for worming your horse.

Questions and Answers

Q. What kind of worms affect horses?

A. There are some 150 different species of parasites that may affect horses. The chief and most dangerous ones are:

Stomach Bots. Larvae of the bot fly which lays its eggs on the legs of horses. They enter the stomach when the horse bites or licks the area.

Ascarids (Large Roundworms). The larval form of the parasite migrates through the bloodstream and lungs. Adult worms irritate the intestines and may cause stoppage and irregularity of the bowels.

Strongyles (Hookworms). They hook onto and suck blood from the intestines.

Pinworms. These irritate the lower bowel and anal region.

Tapeworms. Parasites that form a cluster at the junction of the small and large intestines.

Q. Will the worming drugs I can get in my tack shop control all of these worms?

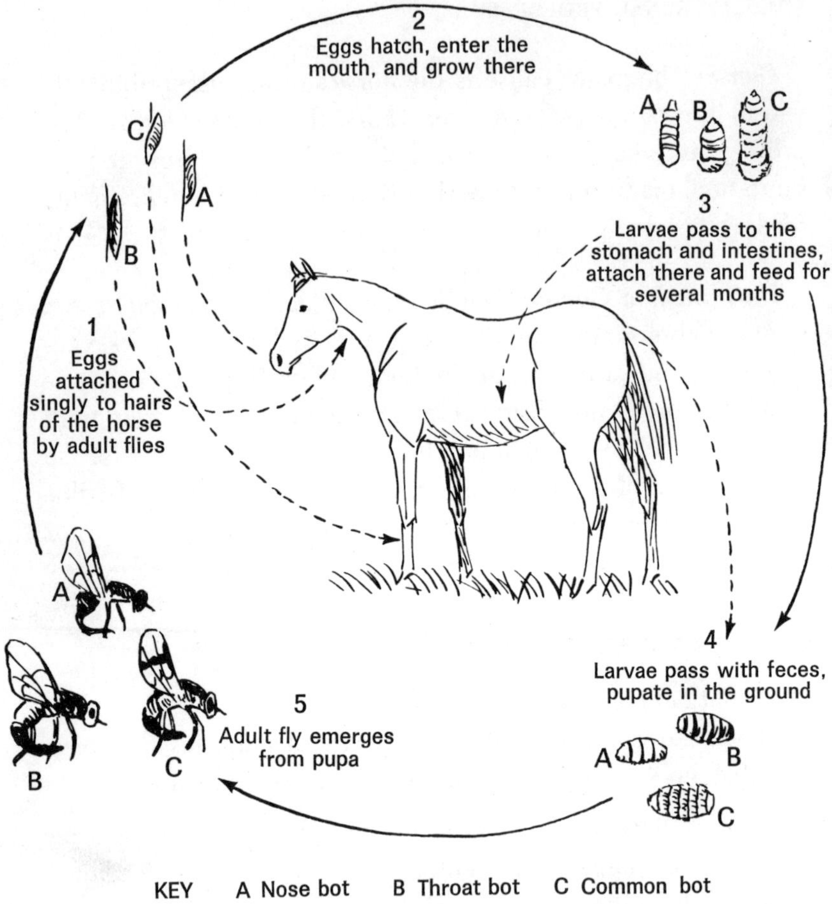

Bot fly cycle

A. No. All the vermifuges developed so far are more specific for some species of parasites than for others. That is why at least once a year you should provide your veterinarian with a sample of your horse's manure so that the kind of worms your horse has, and the degree of infestation, can be determined. It used to be the fashion to worm horses twice a year, in spring and fall. Today's knowledge calls for more frequent worming. Ask your vet.

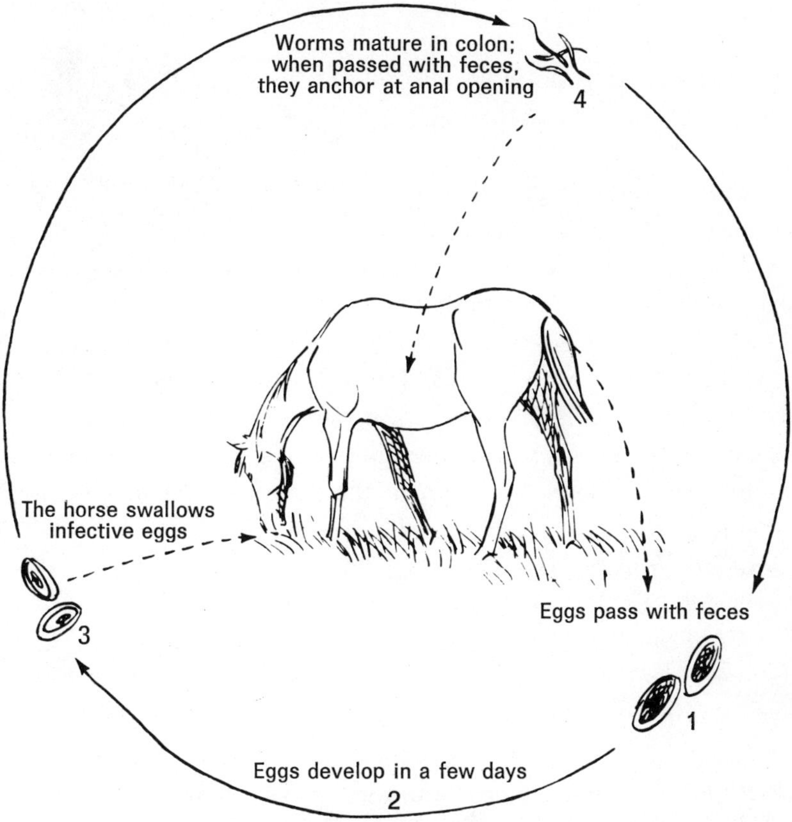

Pinworm cycle

Q. Can worming drugs be dangerous to the horse?

A. Yes. Any drug that destroys parasites is also poisonous to the horse. The dose given must be one that destroys parasites without injuring the animal. Carefully follow the directions on the label and the advice of your veterinarian.

TIE-UP OR AZOTURIA

Tie-up or azoturia is an excessive contraction of muscles caused by an excess of the by-products of muscle activity. The horse's system is not able to throw off these waste products of exercise rapidly enough.

Signs: Hardening of the muscles of the croup and loins, accompanied by a staggering or rolling action, and then a noticeably stiffened gait. The horse exhibits excitability, profuse sweating, and rapid breathing.

Cause: Hard exercise following idleness and heavy feeding. It used to be called "Monday Morning Disease," because it so frequently afflicted workhorses that were given a few days' rest without a reduction of grain in the diet. It is not uncommon today among race horses, other performance horses, and ponies worked off lush spring pasture.

Until the Vet Comes: Stop the animal and remove its tack at the first sign of stiffening behind and the other symptoms. From now on the problem is to keep the horse warm and *to prevent further exertion.* Cover the animal with three or four blankets with emphasis on the croup and loins. If no blankets are available, use your coat. If you can get the horse back to the stall, bed the stall down well. Wet the contents of a pound box of baking soda with just enough water to allow you to administer as much as possible to the horse with a drench bottle or syringe. Put a handful of baking soda in a bucket of warm water for the horse to drink. Do not feed oats or corn. Instead, prepare a mash from bran or barley. Add two handfuls of bicarbonate of soda to the feed. Until the vet comes you want to keep the horse warm and quiet.

Questions and Answers

Q. How do I prepare a mash?
A. For one horse, four to six good double handfuls of bran and

about a tablespoon of common salt make an ordinary mash. You may add barley or linseed meal. Add enough boiling water to dampen. Stir until it is well mixed and cover the bucket with a sack. After steaming for about 15 minutes, it should be cool enough for the horse to eat.

COLDS

Colds in horses are much like those in humans. They are also considered to be due to a virus.

Signs: Sneezing is often one of the first symptoms. The horse may be slightly feverish and off his feed. There is a discharge from the nose, and the eyes water. If the temperature does not subside in a few days, call the vet. Although colds are a minor ailment, there may be secondary difficulties.

Cause: Heavily worked animals exposed to damp and chilly conditions are particularly susceptible. The horse may catch a cold from other horses. Using a common water trough, bucket,

Caring for the sick horse

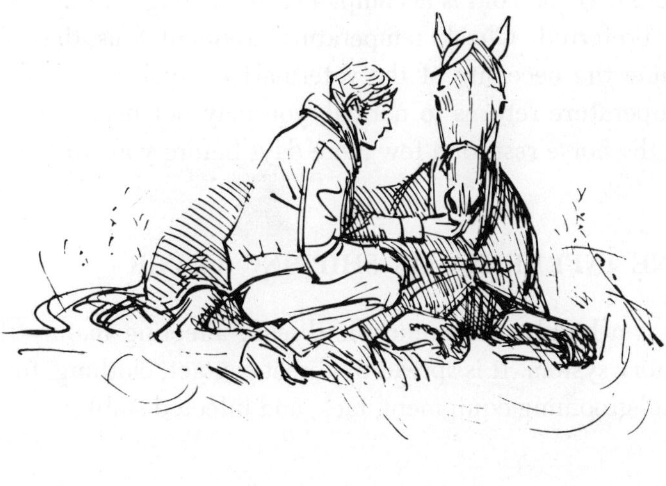

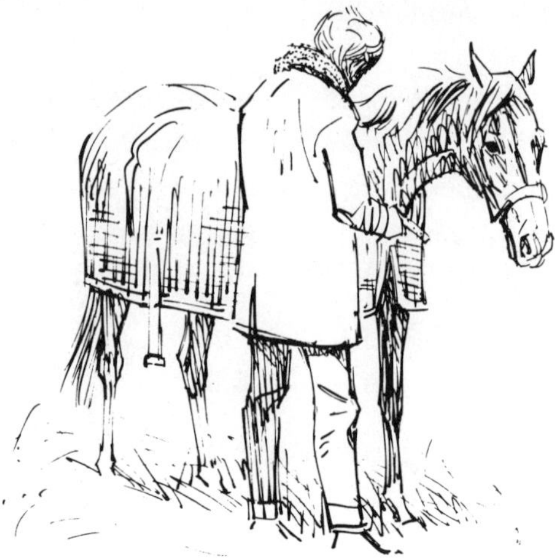

Keep the sick horse warm.

or manger can bring about a cold. Direct contact is not needed to contract a viral infection.

Until the Vet Comes: Put the horse in a well-ventilated but draft-free stall. Blanket it well. Feed warm bran mashes, and let the horse have all the water it wants to drink. Change the water frequently. Administer inhalations medicated with a sprinkling of oil of eucalyptus or Friar's Balsam (available at your drugstore). If the cold is accompanied by a cough, Friar's Balsam is preferred. Check temperature frequently as this will determine the necessity of the veterinarian's making a call. If the temperature returns to normal, you may not need the vet. But let the horse rest for a few more days before you work him.

EQUINE INFLUENZA OR SHIPPING FEVER

This is a highly communicable disease affecting mainly the respiratory system. It is spread by direct contact, clothing, food, bedding, grooming equipment, tack, and infected stables.

Signs: They occur suddenly, with a temperature of 103° to 106° F. which lasts for about three days. There is depression and a loss of appetite, rapid breathing, cough, and frequently a watery nasal discharge. The mucous membrane of the eyelid has a reddish color tinged with yellow. Often the nasal discharge becomes thick and yellow. The legs, muzzle, and belly may be swollen.

Cause: When horses congregate as they do at horse shows, trail rides, training stables, and race tracks, the chances of respiratory infection greatly increase. At one's own stable, the infection may be introduced by a new horse. Influenza is caused by the horse's eating or breathing in some of the body discharges, particularly the nasal and bowel discharges, of a diseased horse.

Until the Vet Comes: Isolate the horse in a roomy stall. Keep it warm, but allow it to have plenty of fresh air and sunshine. During cold weather, keep the patient well blanketed, with legs bandaged. Give plenty of water, changing it frequently. Try to induce the animal to eat by the frequent offering of small amounts of soft food with tidbits. Steam the head frequently with medicated vapor.

Questions and Answers

Q. What do you mean by tidbits in the horse's feed?
A. A handful of moist brown sugar, or molasses, or sliced carrots or apples added to a mash. The important thing is to get the horse to eat something to maintain its strength. Equine influenza is a very wasting disease.

Q. Does equine influenza lead to complications?
A. It can, and it also can be fatal. Complications can lead to

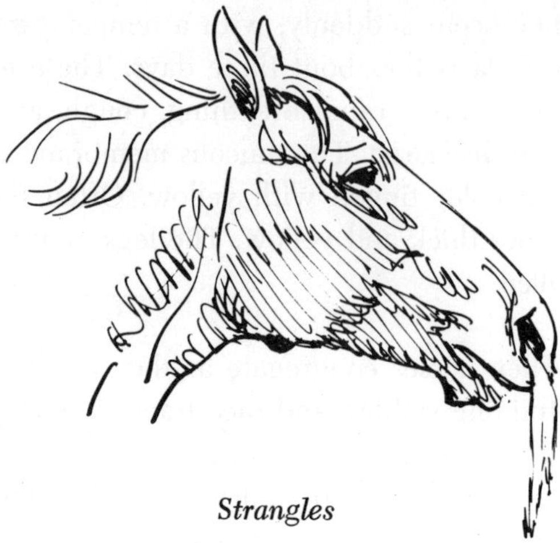

Strangles

permanent respiratory trouble. That is why it is important to call the veterinarian.

STRANGLES

Strangles or equine distemper is an acutely contagious disease of the nose and throat. It is a bacterial disease that most frequently attacks young horses.

Signs: Noticeable dullness and apathy, a rise in temperature, usually to between 103° and 105° F., and loss of appetite. A thin, watery discharge from the nostrils will turn into a thicker, yellowish discharge. Hot and painful swelling can be felt between the jaws. The swelling usually develops into an abcess after a week, and bursts. In more serious cases, abcesses develop in other parts of the body.

Cause: Contact with a diseased animal, contaminated stalls, hay, bedding, buckets, or tack.

Until the Vet Comes: Isolate the horse. Let the patient have plenty of fresh air and sunshine, but protect him from drafts. Blanket and bandage according to the weather. Give inhalations of oil of eucalyptus or Friar's Balsam. Clean out the nose tenderly with Vap-O-Rub on soft cotton. Feed soft and easily digested food. Tempt the patient to eat with sprinkled tidbits on the feed or mixed with the feed.

CONGESTION OF THE LUNGS

This is due to an abnormal quantity of blood in the lungs.

Signs: Exaggerated breathing, heaving flanks and chest wall, weak pulse, eye membranes a dull bluish color, and temperature that may rise as high as 106° F. The horse will stand with legs outstretched, extending the head and neck. He may break into a cold sweat.

Cause: The cause may be a bacterial invasion, irritating chemicals such as medicine, or exposure to bad weather.

Until the Vet Comes: If you are out riding, remove the saddle, loosen throat latch of bridle, turn the horse's head to the wind, and throw your coat over his back. Keep him still for at least half an hour. Lead him to the stable.

Put the patient in a well-ventilated stall, keep him warm, and feed laxative and nutritious food. Get the veterinarian there as soon as possible.

PNEUMONIA

This inflammation of the lungs is probably due to an invasion of virulent organisms. It frequently follows influenza or strangles.

Signs: Breathing becomes hurried and difficult, and there is noticeable dullness and loss of appetite. The temperature rises and the animal reveals muscular weakness and a staggering gait. There may be a cough, a nasal discharge, and attacks of shivering, and the horse is not likely to lie down.

Cause: Causes are the same as in congestion. Senility, anemia, or general disability are all contributing factors.

Until the Vet Comes: Keep the animal warm and well blanketed in a box stall that allows for plenty of fresh air. Medicated inhalations may be given (oil of eucalyptus, Friar's Balsam), and the bowels should be kept open with four tablespoons of Epsom Salts in the drinking water. This is a serious disease and it is most important that the veterinarian arrive soon.

PLEURISY

Signs: The horse will be off his feed and may show colicky symptoms. The animal appears stiff. He is not inclined to move and will groan if forced. Breathing is fast, and flank and abdomen work excessively and noticeably. There may be a short painful cough and discharge from the eyes and nose.

Cause: Causes are the same as those that bring about pneumonia. Pleurisy can also be the result of a wound in the wall of the chest.

Until the Vet Comes: First aid is the same as in pneumonia. Keep the patient in a well-ventilated stall, but keep him warm with blankets and bandages. Rub the chest wall with a counter irritant. Four tablespoons of Epsom Salts should be given in the drinking water.

CONGESTION OF THE KIDNEYS

This is a kidney condition, the treatment of which depends entirely on the veterinarian's diagnosis.

Signs: The first signs may be a large amount of pale urine passed, a staggery gait, and stiffness over the loins. Loss of condition may be quite noticeable and there may be constipation.

Cause: Failure of the kidneys to excrete impure substances that have entered the blood as a result of illness or feeding poor quality hay and grain. Injuries in the area of the loins, or chill, may also cause the condition.

Until the Vet Comes: Keep the horse warmly blanketed and bandaged, and keep the patient at rest. Feed bran mashes. Adding linseed in some form to the mashes will help.

STAGGERS

This is a condition similar to fainting in human beings.

Signs: Attacks generally occur when a horse is being ridden. The horse will stop, sway, stagger, and fall to the ground unconscious. The attacks last about five minutes.

Cause: Staggers is due to:

Defective circulation, caused by a weak heart or undue restraint of tack.
Digestive problems as a result of incorrect feeding.
Congestion of the brain.
Worms.

Until the Vet Comes: Remove all possible causes of restraint, such as saddle and bridle. Apply cold water to the head.

THUMPS

Thumps are spasms of the diaphragm.

Signs: Abrupt and violent beating of the heart causing spasmodic jerking in the belly and flanks. Usually a thumping sound can be heard quite distinctly.

Cause: Thumps may be due to an organic disease of the heart, digestive disorder, overexertion, or excitement. Overwork, or fast work in hot weather, with an animal not in condition, is a common cause.

Until the Vet Comes: If you are riding the horse, stop and reduce the animal's temperature by sponging with cool water. Lead the horse back to the stable at a walk. Put him in a quiet, comfortable stall away from anything that may tend to excite him. Feed bran mashes and easily digested foods.

5

SKIN DISEASES

CONTAGIOUS SKIN DISEASES: Ringworm — Mange — Lice — Itchy Tail or Mane
NONCONTAGIOUS SKIN DISEASES: Humour — Nettlerash or Hives — Cracked Heels and Mud Fever

Skin diseases are divided into two groups—those which arise from infection by either germs or parasites, and those due to causes other than infection.

Of the infectious diseases, the ones most likely to be contagious are ringworm and mange, and the one most often met with by horseowners is itchy tail or mane.

CONTAGIOUS SKIN DISEASES

RINGWORM

This is the same skin disease that sometimes afflicts people. It is contagious to human beings.

Signs: First signs are raised circular patches of hair, generally on the neck and shoulders. Shortly after these appear, the skin is left bare, showing an almost white crust.

Cause: Ringworm is caused by a fungus, a parasite in the skin. Winter and spring are the seasons in which it is most likely to occur.

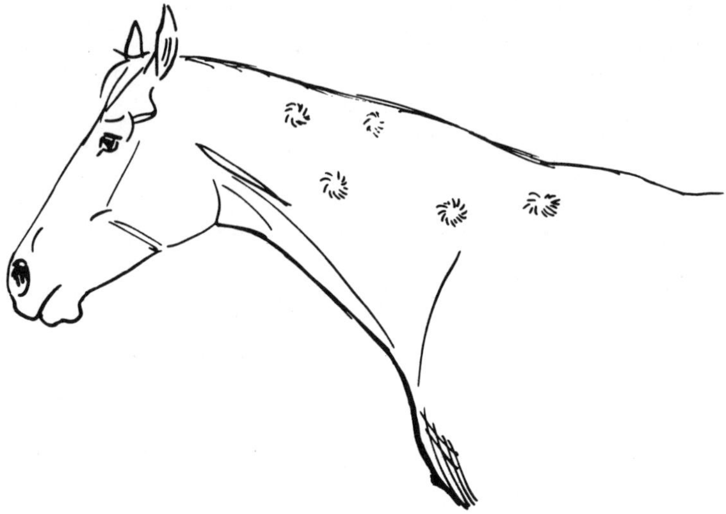

Ringworm

Until the Vet Comes: Because of the contagious nature of ringworm, isolate the horse immediately and disinfect all gear and tack. The ringworm patches should be washed with a warm solution of washing soda applied with a stiff brush. When the patches are dry, work iodine well into them. This is first aid and only the first step. All cases of ringworm require veterinary attention.

MANGE

Mange is due to a mite or parasite too small to be seen by the naked eye. There are three types or forms of mange. The important thing to understand is that, in any form, mange is very infectious and contagious.

Signs: Intense irritation of the skin. Affected parts then become thickened and wrinkled, and the hair eventually falls off, leaving the skin covered with small crusts.

Until the Vet Comes: Isolate the animal at once. Disinfect all contact materials and put the horse on a diet low in concentrates. Call the veterinarian, because mange is another disease of the skin that requires skilled professional attention.

LICE

Lice is an infectious skin disease commonly met with when horses are on pasture. The long hairs of mane and tail pick up the eggs while the horse is grazing.

Signs: The parasites are usually found around the ears, along the neck, close to the mane, at the points of the shoulder, and at the buttocks near the root of the tail. Lice give rise to a blotchy appearance of the coat and, since they are blood-sucking animals, are harmful to the horse's condition. They are generally present when a horse is seen to rub against convenient objects. Examination shows lice and nits on the horse.

Lice

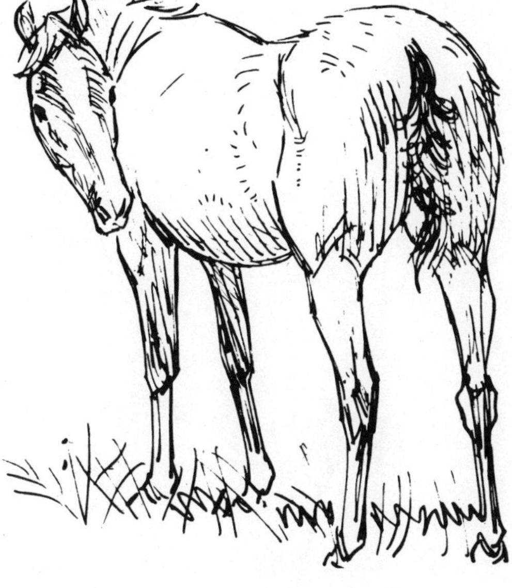

Cause: The most common louse found on the horse is equipped with a boring and sucking apparatus and is scientifically referred to as a haematopinus.

Until the Vet Comes: Groom the animal thoroughly and disinfect the grooming materials. Louse control requires direct application of insecticides to the skin of the animal. Do not treat this disease with disinfectants. They have no value against lice and only blister the skin. Consult your veterinarian.

ITCHY TAIL OR MANE

This is either a parasitic disease or the result of a disordered condition of the blood.

Signs: The horse will rub its tail or mane on solid objects, causing the hair to drop out.

Cause: Worms may be the cause as well as external parasites.

Itchy tail

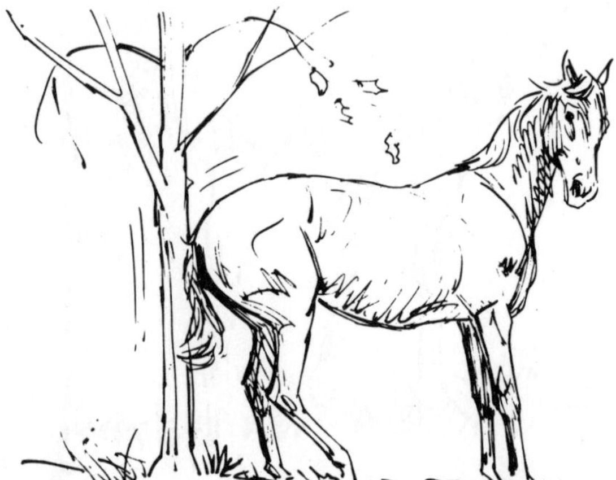

Until the Vet Comes: Wash the affected parts with a mild solution of disinfectant and put the horse on a low concentrate diet. Application of soothing oil may relieve itchiness. If the condition persists, consult the veterinarian.

Noncontagious Skin Diseases

These diseases are frequently due to faulty feeding as well as external conditions such as weather and stable management.

HUMOUR

This is a not uncommon, pimply condition of the skin.

Signs: Pimples which may occur on almost any part of the animal's body.

Cause: Humour commonly occurs when a horse is put on concentrates to a greater degree than it has been accustomed.

Until the Vet Comes: Keep the bowels well open by feeding a laxative diet. Cut down on concentrates. The pimples often disappear as quickly as they arrive. You may not need the vet.

NETTLERASH OR HIVES

This skin disorder is more scientifically known as Urticaria. It is not uncommon, and not much of a problem.

Signs: Round elevations or swellings appear suddenly on the skin at various parts of the animal's body. These swellings are usually raised areas varying in size from that of a pea to several inches across.

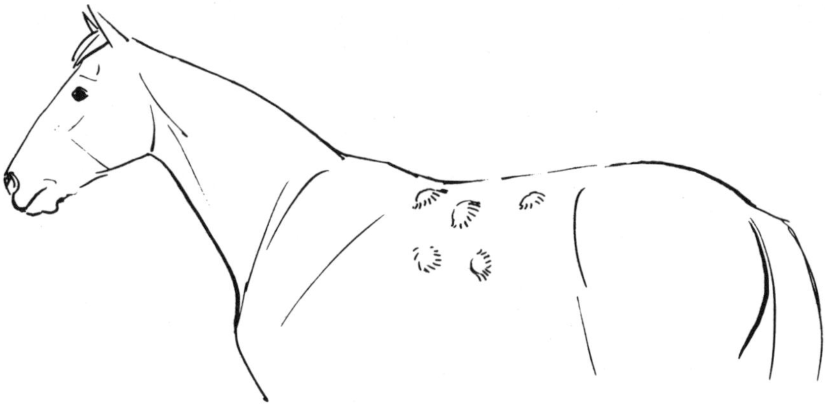

Nettlerash or hives

Cause: An idle horse still getting a working diet is subject to this skin disease. Insect bites may be another cause.

Until the Vet Comes: Slow down on concentrates and feed a more laxative diet. The chances are you won't have to call the veterinarian. In most instances this condition disappears spontaneously.

CRACKED HEELS AND MUD FEVER

These conditions are similar to chapped hands in humans and are an inflammation of the skin on the heels, legs, and sometimes the belly.

Signs: The skin cracks and forms deep creases; there may be a slight, greasy seepage; and frequently the legs become stocked and swollen.

Cause: Weak circulation, blood disorder, or a lymphatic constitution may be predisposing causes. More immediate causes may be mud and wetness, and frequently washing the horse's legs after work and not drying them. Washing the legs and heels removes the natural oil and leaves the skin dry and brittle.

Until the Vet Comes: Wash the heels with hot water and medicated soap and dry thoroughly. Apply a zinc ointment to the area and cut down on rich food such as corn. Keep the horse out of the mud, keep the stable clean, and stop any cracks that admit drafts. In view of the area affected, you will want the vet to have a look and perhaps give a dose of tetanus antitoxin and a course of antibiotics.

6

INJURIES

Tetanus — Minor Injuries — Puncture Wounds — Deep Wounds — Injuries That Do Not Break the Skin

TETANUS

Tetanus is not really an injury but rather the horrible result of an injury. Any wound may permit the introduction of *Bacillus tetani* and cause tetanus, even one as small as a pinprick invisible to the eye.

Signs: A general stiffening of the limbs, and the horse will stand with nose and tail stretched out. The temperature rises to between 103° and 105° F. The horse will be in a nervous state, and sudden noise or movement will cause every muscle to tauten.

Be sure your horse is properly immunized against tetanus. If your horse should become afflicted due to lack of immunization or regular booster shots, there is nothing you can do until the vet comes.

MINOR INJURIES

Horses are forever getting minor nicks and cuts, particularly on the legs. In most instances, they are of no consequence. Apply a good wound preparation, of which there are many available to the horseowner. Many horsemen are particularly partial to preparations containing nitrofurazone. These come in both ointment form and aerosol cans.

PUNCTURE WOUNDS

Punctures are dangerous in that they may be small and overlooked. They present the danger of healing from the surface and enclosing pus which eventually demands that the wound be reopened. Puncture wounds are also a perfect environment for tetanus organisms.

DEEP WOUNDS

One of the major problems with deep wounds is stopping the bleeding. This is not so difficult if the bleeding is only from the veins. Applying plenty of cold water will stop that bleeding.

However, if the blood is a bright scarlet and issues in spurts from the wound, the bleeding is arterial and the cut should be bathed continuously in cold water, or a pressure bandage should be applied. Call for veterinary aid immediately.

After bleeding has stopped, the wound should be cleansed and mild medication applied.

INJURIES THAT DO NOT BREAK THE SKIN

Injuries such as bruises and abrasions, and those resulting from kicks or blows, respond well to cold applications, as cold relieves pain and prevents or reduces swelling. Irritated areas caused by tack—saddle, girth, or cinch sores—are also aided by cold treatment. This, however, is layman's first aid. If any injury is serious, or becomes infected, call the veterinarian.

7

PREVENTION: SOME ABC'S OF HORSE HEALTH MANAGEMENT

A. *Shots.* Immunologic procedures (vaccination, "shots") are routine in the control of livestock disease. Make sure you have them regularly for your horse *and keep a record.* Shots are invaluable, but their value is also relative. The value of immunologic procedures may be overcome by extensive exposure to a disease, contact with an unusually powerful strain of an infecting agent, or stress caused by poor stable management. Shots are no cure-all and should be accompanied by good horse-management measures.

On a yearly basis, your animals should be immunized against tetanus and the strains of equine encephalomyelitis for which there are vaccines. If you intend to show or attend events at which there are large gatherings of horses, get flu shots (rhinopneumonitis vaccination). If rabies is a problem in your area, get shots for rabies. At any rate, yearly protection against tetanus and equine encephalomyelitis is a must. These are shots you cannot do without.

B. *External Parasites.* Just as internal parasites (worms) are a menace to a horse's health and condition, so are external parasites (flies, mosquitoes, lice, ticks, and so on). External parasites are a great annoyance to the horse and during the fly season may cause considerable loss of weight and condition. Furthermore, insects are disease carriers. For example, equine encephalomyelitis (sleeping sickness) and equine infectious anemia (swamp fever) are both transmitted by insects. The

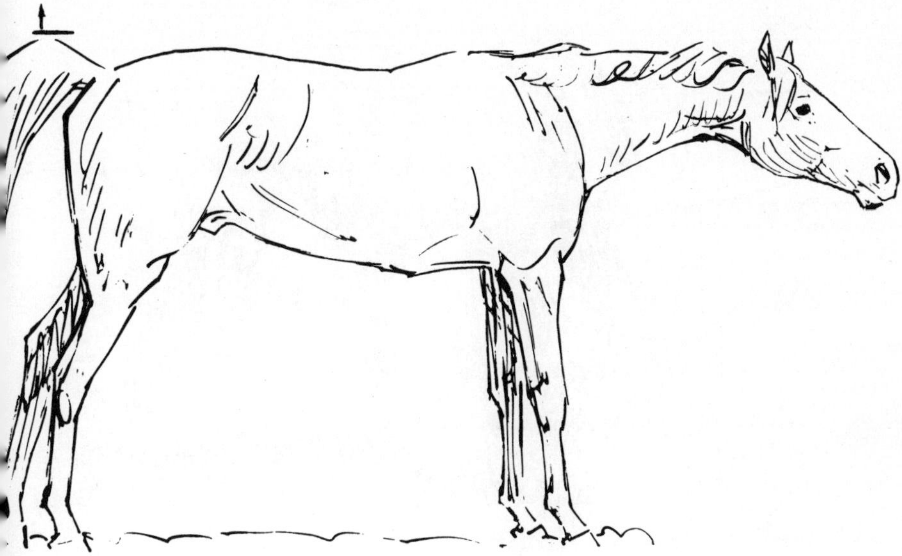

Tetanus symptoms

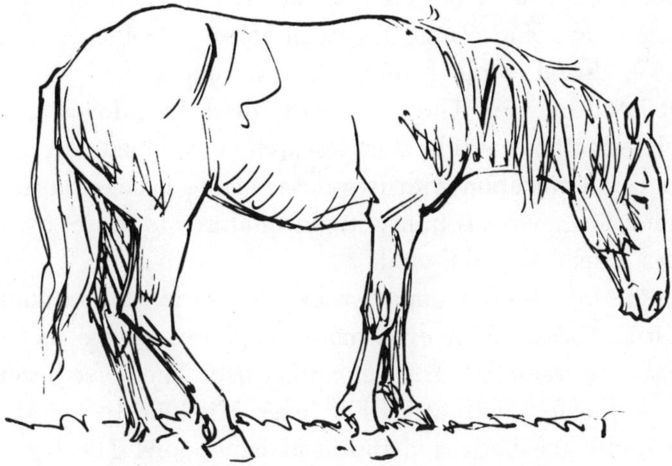

Equine encephalomyelitis (sleeping sickness)

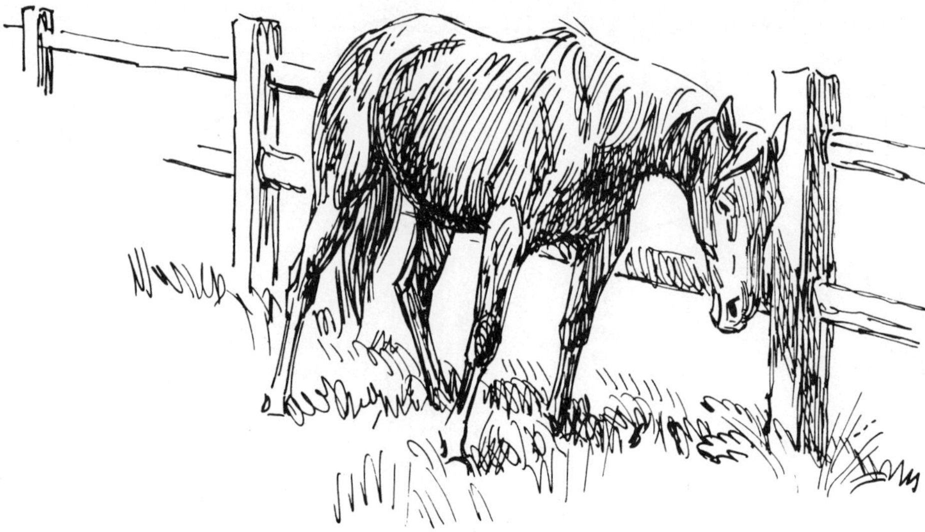

Equine infectious anemia (swamp fever)

only measures to be taken against both diseases are preventative. That is why they are included here.

The cause of equine encephalomyelitis and a vaccine for the nerve disease were discovered by the veterinarian Dr. Karl F. Meyer while director of The George William Hooper foundation in California. Horsemen in the San Joaquin Valley had become aware of a strange disease of horses. The horses became feverish, dozed while leaning against fences, and stumbled about in odd circles. They frequently died. Dr. Meyer and his associates, after considerable research, developed a vaccine. Annual immunization with two doses of the vaccine is recommended. Since virus is transmitted from birds to horses by mosquitoes, insect control is vital.

Equine infectious anemia (swamp fever) is another dangerous virus disease made even more dangerous by the fact that no means of treatment or vaccination exists. The horse becomes weak, depressed, with attacks of fever. His hind feet shift forward under the body and the head hangs low. The legs and lower chest wall may swell. However, a horse may have swamp fever, or be a carrier, and yet show no outward signs of the disease. The "Coggins Test" determines whether an animal is afflicted. Your only preventive measure against equine infectious anemia is insect control.

To control insects:

Use screens and good sanitation methods to eliminate breeding places.
Drain low swampy areas.
During the fly season turn horses out at night rather than during the day.
Use insecticides in your stable and on your horses, *but carefully read and follow directions.*

C. ***Man-made Hazards.*** Horses have an uncanny knack for injuring themselves. Keep your eyes open for injury-producing hazards and eliminate them.

Do away with sharp protruding objects.

Horses use the "buddy system" to keep off flies.

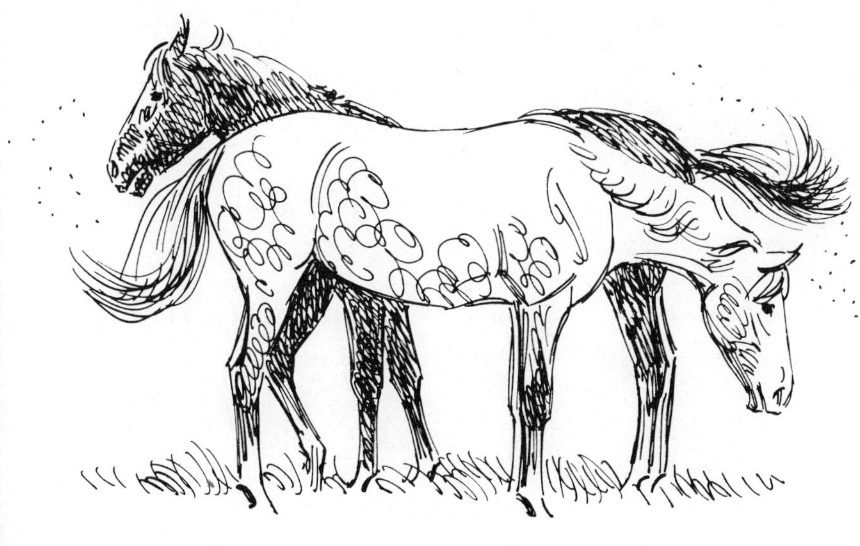

Get rid of waterers and feeders that are worn out.

Don't leave tools, shovels, or rakes around where they can cause injury.

When tying a horse, tie him to a solid object with a slip knot. Never tie a horse to anything movable.

Make sure your fencing presents no hazards. Never use barbed wire!

Halters can present problems. When turning a horse out, either remove the halter or make sure it will break readily if it gets caught on something.

D. ***Feeding and Watering.*** There is an old proverb: "It is the eye of the owner that makes a horse fat." It is your eye that

Never tie a horse to a movable object.

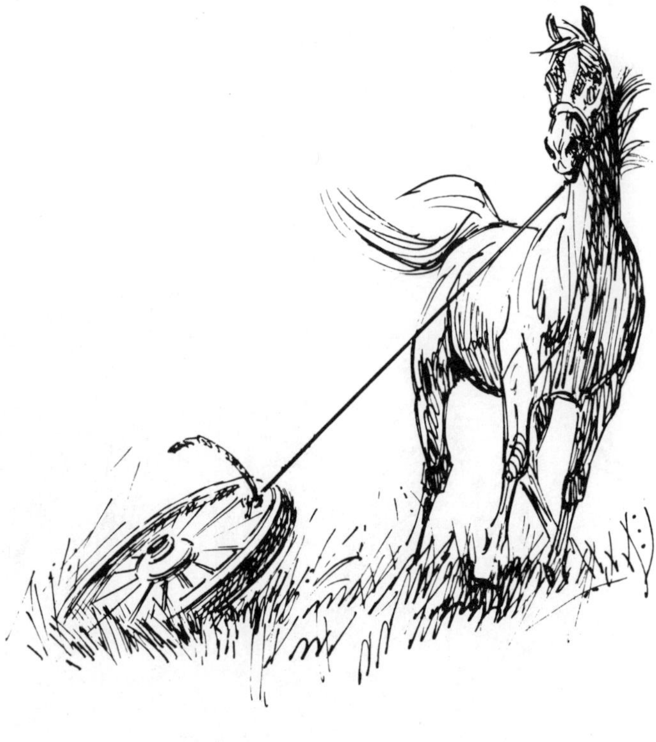

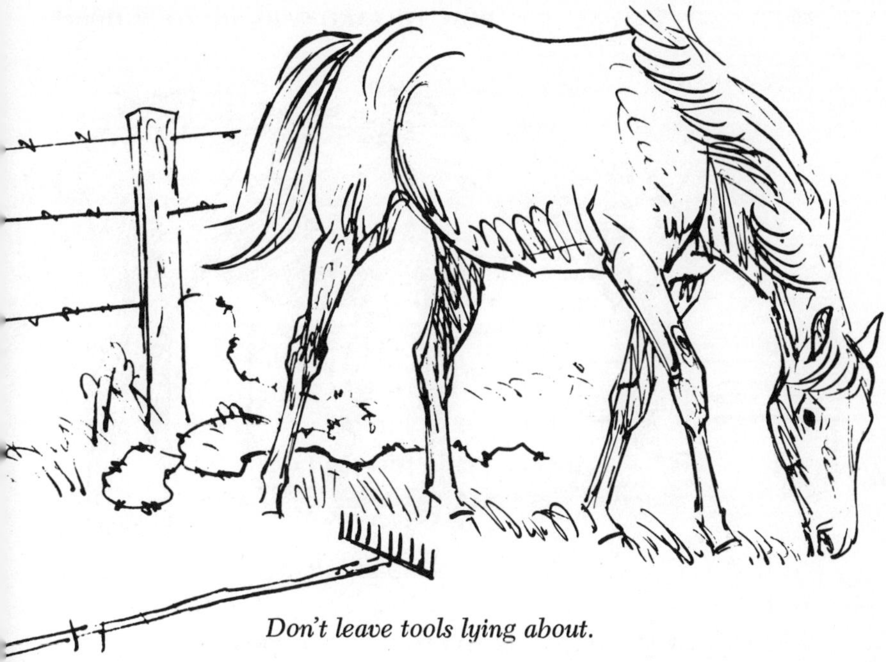

Don't leave tools lying about.

Halters can cause injuries.

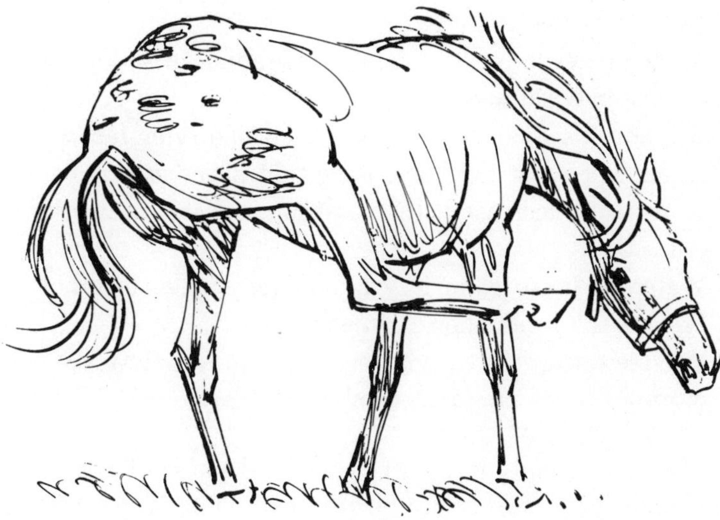

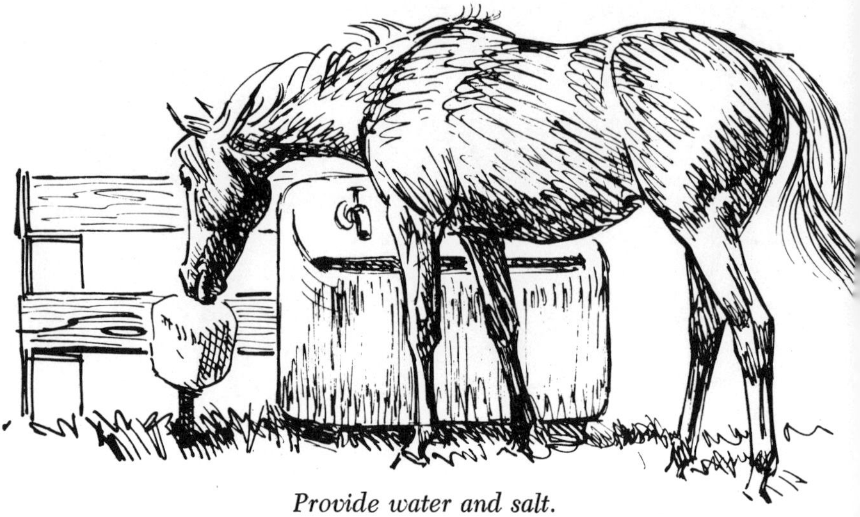

Provide water and salt.

tells you if you are feeding and watering properly.

Feed little but often. Never overtax the horse's digestive system by overfeeding at any one feeding.

Feed regularly. Horses become accustomed to a certain schedule of feeding. If the routine is not followed, they fret and get nervous.

Any changes in feeding should be gradual. A sudden feeding change may cause colic.

Balance the amount of grain or concentrates fed with the amount of work the horse is getting. Decrease concentrates as work is decreased. Increase concentrates as work is increased.

Water the horse frequently and liberally unless he is hot.

Provide salt for the horse's free choice.

Provide only clean, bright feeds for the horse. Musty, dusty, or moldy feeds can cause trouble.

E. *Teeth.* Probably the most overlooked phase of horse health management is care of the horse's teeth. This may be because ordinarily the horse's teeth are no great problem. Tooth decay is uncommon in horses. A horse's teeth are generally healthy if the horse is getting a balanced diet and has a normal jaw. Toothache is rare in horses, but it can occur. The problem is indicated when the horse is eating or drinking, suddenly stops chewing, and opens its mouth and throws its head to one side. The remedy is extraction.

However, in spite of the fact that a horse's teeth seldom present problems, if your horse loses condition, the chances are the problem is either worms or inadequate care of the teeth. Due to the fact that the upper and lower molars do not cover each other entirely, irregular growth of the edges occurs and these often need attention. The horse's teeth are vital for proper mastication, and therefore the digestion of food. The process of removing irregular tooth growth by filing down sharp projections that interfere with chewing or damage tongue and cheeks is called floating. This is a simple job for the veterinarian. Have him check your horse's teeth at least once a year.

F. *Conditioning.* The horse that is asked to perform safely as an athlete needs to be conditioned as an athlete. With the horse, as with humans, the muscles must be fatigued to an increasing degree daily over a long period of time in order to build en-

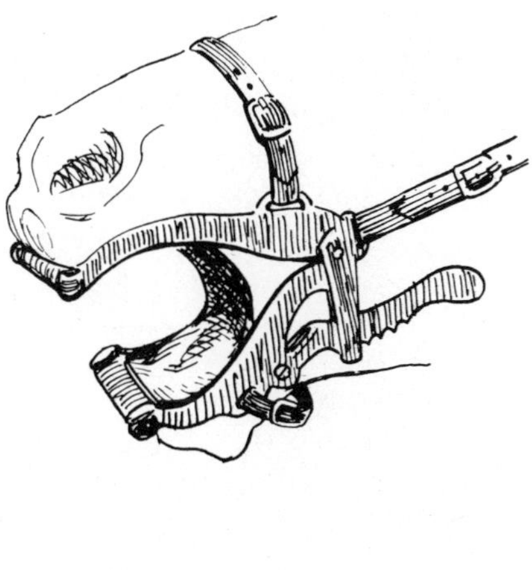

The speculum, an instrument used by the vet to keep a horse's mouth open while its teeth are being floated

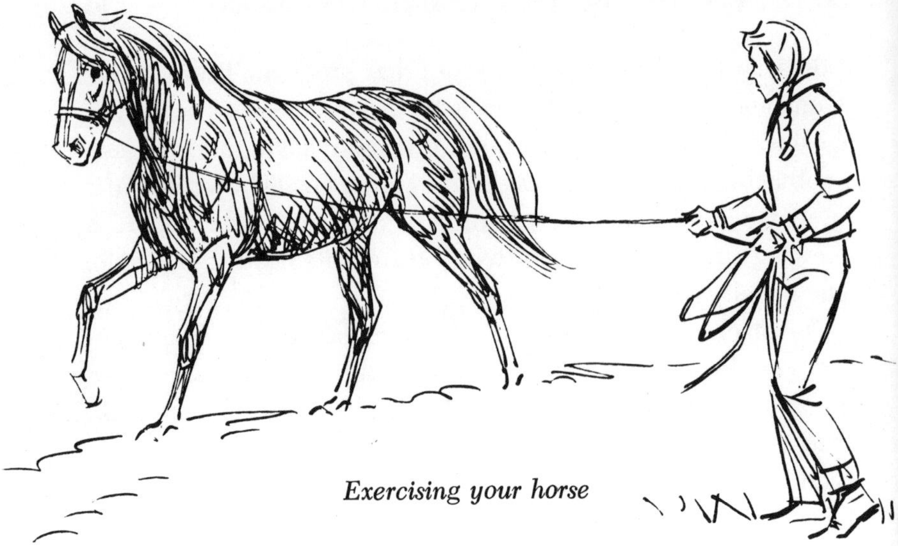

Exercising your horse

durance and make joint articulation stronger and more stable.

The horseowner should have a definite program in mind, first to build muscle and strengthen tendons, and then to develop heart and wind. The owner should be familiar with the major muscles of the horse and work out exercises that can develop them—for instance the neck muscles, which are very important. The neck muscles can be developed by walking the horse with its head well up for short periods, later for longer periods and then at the trot. Thigh and loin muscles can be developed by climbing steep inclines; shoulder muscles and hocks by going down such inclines. The hocks are also strengthened by stopping when going down an incline.

There is no short cut to conditioning. A soft horse should be given very slow work for a period of weeks. A horse in poor condition when pushed too quickly will probably damage its legs. Trying to rush condition into the animal may also permanently affect its wind.

One thing that aids conditioning, however, is the terrain the horse is ridden over. Riding up and down hill at a strong walk, and later at a trot, not only builds the horse's muscle but also strengthens wind. All conditioning is a balancing act between exertion needed to build muscle and wind and the resulting stress that could lead to tearing down joints.

G. ***Until the Vet Comes.*** List the questions you want to ask the veterinarian. How many times have you seen the tailgate of your veterinarian's station wagon vanish from your driveway as you suddenly realized that the one question you thought was uppermost in your mind was never asked? Usually when the veterinarian arrives in response to your call he is there to deal with a specific problem. There is not much time for talk. Be prepared.

Be ready to ask him as he treats your animal:

How does the horse look to you?
How are his teeth?

Conditioning your horse

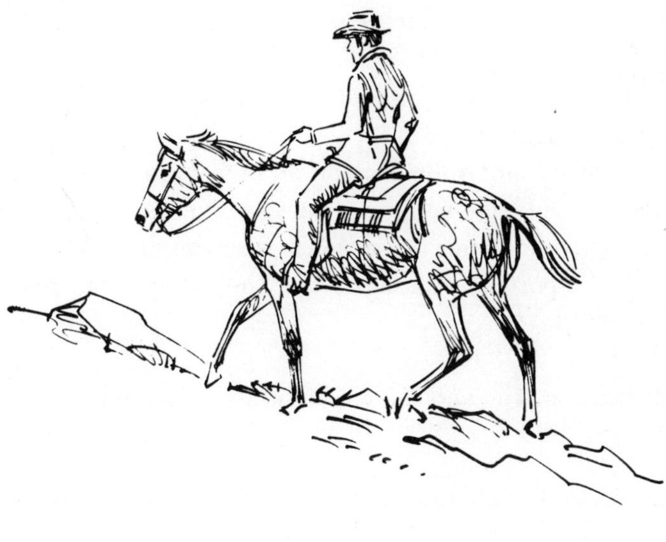

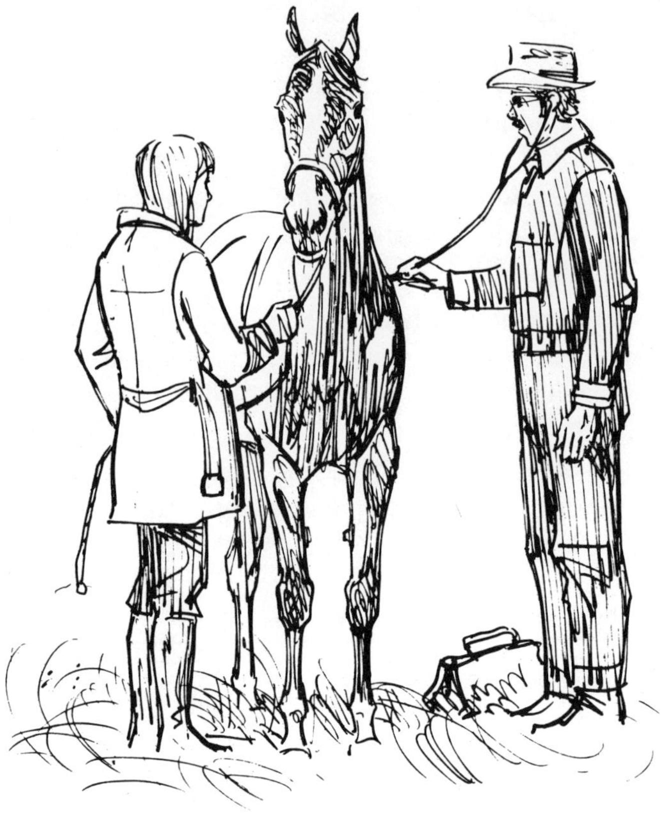

You and the vet are a team.

What do you think of his feet and the way he is shod? Do you have any suggestions?
What am I doing right, Doctor, and what am I doing wrong?
And, you will have your own questions, more directly related both to you and your horse. Make sure you don't forget them on that important occasion when the veterinarian responds to your call.

H. ***Remember.*** You and the veterinarian are a team.

INDEX

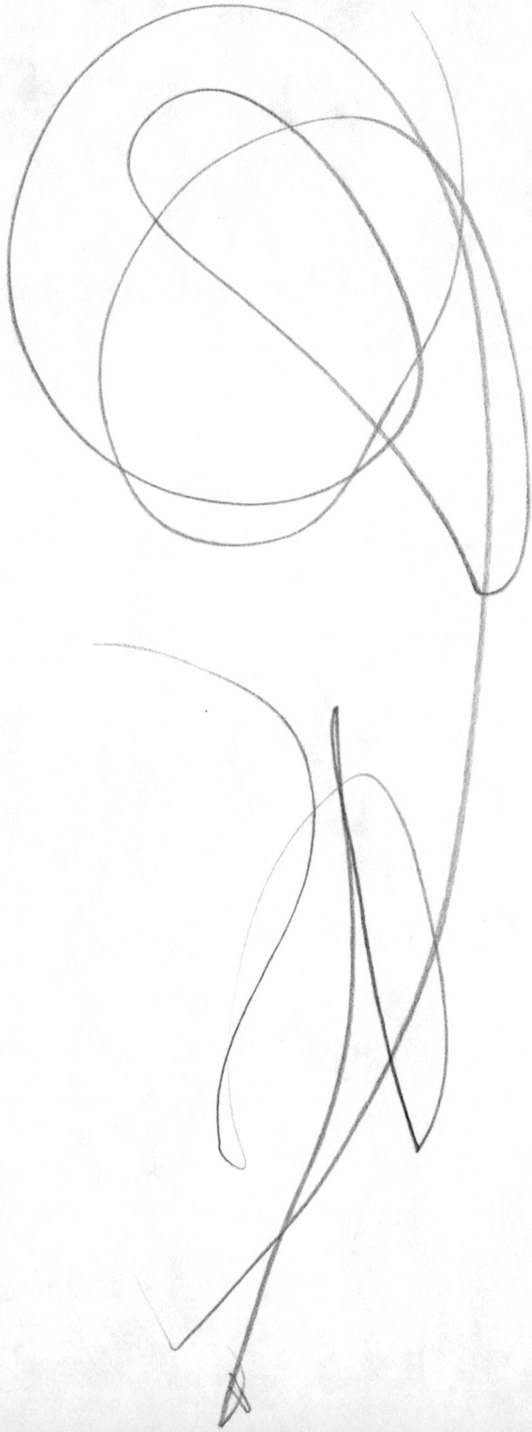

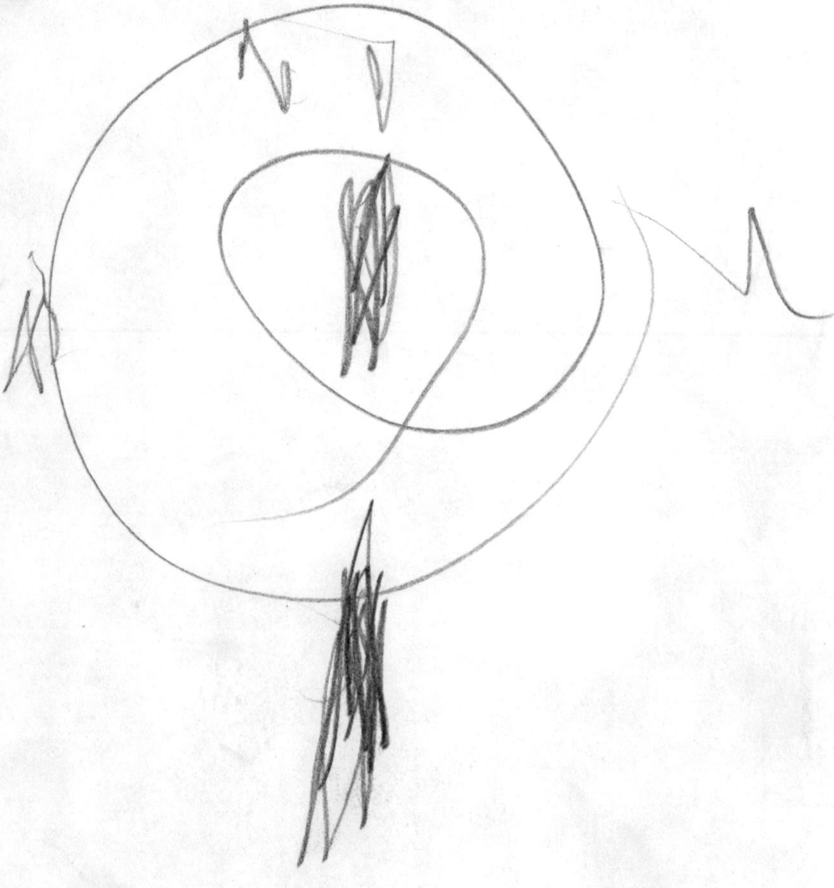